T0186232

Cognitive-Behavioral Treatment
of Irritable Bowel Syndrome

TREATMENT MANUALS FOR PRACTITIONERS
David H. Barlow, *Editor*

Cognitive-Behavioral Treatment of Irritable Bowel Syndrome

The Brain–Gut Connection

BRENDA B. TONER
ZINDEL V. SEGAL
SHELAGH D. EMMOTT
DAVID MYRAN

Series Editor's Note by David H. Barlow
Foreword by Douglas A. Drossman

THE GUILFORD PRESS
New York   London

This book is printed on acid-free paper.

Last digit is print number: 9 8 7 6 5 4 3

Library of Congress Cataloging-in-Publication Data

Cognitive-behavioral treatment of irritable bowel syndrome:
the brain–gut connection / Brenda B. Toner ... [et al.];
foreword by Douglas A. Drossman.
    p. ; cm. — (Treatment manuals for practitioners)
  Includes bibliographical references and index.
  ISBN 1-57230-135-X (hardcover : alk. paper)
   1. Irritable colon–Psychosomatic aspects. 2. Cognitive
therapy. I. Toner, Brenda B. II. Series
[DNLM: 1. Colonic Diseases, Functional–therapy.
2. Behavior Therapy. 3. Cognitive Therapy.
WI 520 C676 1999]
RC862.I77 C64 1999
616.3'42–dc21   99-042921

To our families,
for their continued love and support

About the Authors

Brenda B. Toner, PhD, is Head of the Women's Mental Health Program and Associate Professor in the Department of Psychiatry at the University of Toronto. She is also Head of the Women's Mental Health Research Section at the Centre for Addiction and Mental Health in Toronto. Dr. Toner has published numerous articles on psychosocial issues and treatment of functional gastrointestinal disorders and frequently gives workshops and presentations to health care professionals working with individuals with irritable bowel syndrome. She also sits on the Advisory Board of the International Foundation for Functional Gastrointestinal Disorders.

Zindel V. Segal, PhD, is Head of the Cognitive Behaviour Therapy Unit at the Centre for Addiction and Mental Health in Toronto. He is also Professor in the Departments of Psychiatry and Psychology and Head of the Psychotherapy Research for Psychotherapy Program in the Department of Psychiatry at the University of Toronto. The author of numerous articles on cognitive factors underlying affective disorder, Dr. Segal is also an associate editor of *Cognitive Therapy and Research* and serves on the editorial board of a number of other journals.

Shelagh D. Emmott, PhD, is a clinical psychologist who specializes in the cognitive-behavioral treatment of irritable bowel syndrome. Her clinical interests and experiences have focused on conditions where psychological issues have been intermeshed with somatic concerns, especially those with a shame component. After a period of public sector consulting and social research, she worked at the Toronto Hospital for several years, using cognitive-behavioral approaches in treating individuals with social phobia and, as staff psychologist in the Immunodeficiency Clinic, people infected with HIV. Currently, she provides therapy for ongoing research studies of clients with irritable bowel syndrome at the Centre for Addiction and Mental Health, Clarke Division, and also is in private practice.

David Myran, MD, is Assistant Professor of Psychiatry at the University of Toronto and Director of the Clarke Crisis Clinic at the Centre for Addiction and Mental Health, where he is also a consultant to the Cognitive Behaviour Therapy Unit. He supervises psychiatric residents in cognitive therapy and has a particular interest in the issues that arise in combining pharmacotherapy with cognitive therapy. Dr. Myran has a significant involvement in geriatric psychiatry and is the coordinator of the Geriatric Psychiatric Community Service at Baycrest Centre for Geriatric Care.

Series Editor's Note

It is much easier to talk about some physical disorders than others. Firmly ensconced among those "hidden" disorders is irritable bowel syndrome (IBS). The reasons why the painful and sometimes disabling symptoms are seldom freely reported are not hard to imagine, since the bloating, gas, and "rumbling stomach" are not pleasant topics of conversation; but the pain and distress would be readily apparent to anyone looking deeply into the eyes of someone suffering from the disorder.

Now Brenda Toner and her colleagues present one of the more sophisticated, empirically supported psychosocial treatments for IBS yet available. Firmly grounded in a biopsychosocial model and recognizing the complex origins of this disorder, this approach covers, in a comprehensive manner, cognitive, emotional, and psychophysiological aspects of this distressing problem. While the embarrassment is distressing enough, the unremitting physical pain associated with IBS can become incapacitating. Since, as the authors point out, the subgroup of patients with particularly severe IBS who seek medical consultation accounts for 12% of primary care cases, it is imperative that all mental health clinicians working in or consulting to primary care or medical settings become aware of this effective and user-friendly treatment program.

DAVID H. BARLOW

Foreword

The understanding and care of persons with irritable bowel syndrome (IBS), the prototype of the functional gastrointestinal disorders, has long been a challenge. Despite the high prevalence of IBS in the community and within clinical practice, knowledge of its pathophysiology and treatment has been limited, and we have come to realize that finding a single "cause" or one specific treatment for this syndrome will be unlikely. This poses a dilemma: The biomedical or disease-based model so entrenched in Western society relies on structural or biochemical abnormalities to define the existence of a medical condition, but for IBS, much like other "functional somatic syndromes" (e.g., fibromyalgia, chronic fatigue syndrome, chronic pain), this model does not fit, so IBS becomes "illegitimate." This "illegitimacy" has considerable impact on patients and their health care providers. When patients with IBS seek medical care for abdominal pain and other gastrointestinal symptoms, the physician may perform a few tests and provide symptomatic relief. But if the symptoms become severe and disabling, or are refractory to usual treatments, the physician and patient may attempt to find the "cause and cure." If tests are done and no underlying cause is determined, the physician may unwittingly amplify the dilemma by indicating that "everything is fine," or by attributing the problem to "nerves." He or she may then advise the patient to "relax," or to see a mental health professional. Now the patient must address the dissonance between his or her personal experience of the physical symptoms and the physician's attribution that "nothing is really wrong" or, possibly by default, that the problem is a psychiatric one.

Recent studies are helping us to redefine IBS as a disorder of neuroenteric function (brain–gut dysfunction) that does not fit into a specific psychiatric or medical condition (Drossman, Whitehead, & Camilleri, 1997). In addition, clinicians and investigators are beginning to move away from the disease-based model to a biopsychosocial understanding of disease and illness. This approach (Engel, 1977; Drossman, 1998) offers a framework for understanding the psychosocial and biological contributors to the symptoms, and for implementing a multicomponent approach to treatment.

I believe that the cognitive-behavioral approach to treating IBS exemplifies this biopsychosocial understanding. It is rational because it directly addresses the maladaptive thoughts and behaviors that emerge from and perpetuate the symptoms of IBS. It is efficient because the treatment approach is highly focused toward achieving what the patient seeks: a means to personally managing the symptoms. It also complements and augments traditional medical care not only by providing ancillary, psychological techniques, but also by moving future responsibility for the care from the health care provider to the patient.

This book, by Brenda Toner, Zindel Segal, Shelagh Emmott, and David Myran, provides the first comprehensive treatise on cognitive-behavioral treatment for IBS. It helps mental health professionals understand the effects of IBS on patients' thinking and behavior and offers specific guidelines for treatment. Beginning with an overview of theoretical and research perspectives, the authors legitimize IBS as a disorder of brain–gut dysfunction. The up-to-date literature review provides an evidence-based elaboration of the theory and in the process helps to remove the stigma of this disorder as "psychiatric."

For physicians or allied health care professionals, the theoretical construct of cognitive-behavioral treatment is clearly presented. It demonstrates and serves to correct the failure of the disease-based biomedical model of illness to explain the symptoms of IBS and their psychological effects. By describing *why* an individual's adherence to this model can lead to selective attention and hypervigilance to bodily symptoms and *how* these factors can lead to a vicious cycle of feelings of ineffectiveness, health care seeking, and social stigmatization, Dr. Toner and colleagues provide health care practitioners with the tools to educate and motivate potential clients to be referred for cognitive-behavioral treatment.

For mental health professionals interested in treating clients with IBS, the authors build upon the key characteristics of cognitive-behavioral treatment: establishing a collaborative therapeutic association that applies questioning rather than interpretation to achieve short-term, problem-based goals and developing an approach that specifically addresses IBS-related cognitions. Common cognitions that typify clients with IBS are presented along with specific guidelines for therapeutic improvement. For example, thoughts such as "Having an intestinal problem is a sign of weakness" or "I am a failure if I embarrass myself in public" are used as examples to develop strategies to ameliorate these maladaptive effects within a context relevant to this clinical population.

A very important and unique contribution of this book is its attention to the social stigma and gender role aspects of IBS. For example, the "passing of gas" is less accepted in Western society for women than for men, and traditionally women may be more conditioned to be helpful to others and feel guilty about taking responsibility for their own needs in the context of their illness. Building upon an emerging body of research on the importance of these factors in the perceptions and behaviors of persons with IBS (much of which is based on Dr. Toner's own published work), a compelling argument is made to incorporate and apply this broader understanding into the treatment approach. For example, Dr. Toner's group has found a strong association between the stereotypically feminine traits of submissiveness and passivity (in conflict with societal expectations of independence and assertiveness) and one's preoccupation with symptoms and tenacious beliefs relating to the seriousness of IBS. Referring to her own studies as well as those of others, Dr. Toner first enlightens us about the importance of these factors in the perceptions and behaviors of women with IBS and then convinces us to adopt two treatment principles in the application of cognitive-behavioral treatment: (1) interpret cognitions and behaviors with respect to not only the physical illness but also social context and gender role, and (2) relabel or reframe "stigmatizing" concepts such as erroneous thinking or cognitive distortions that imply individual psychopathology.

The "Clinical Application" section provides a comprehensive set of treatment recommendations for the therapist. Beginning with an appropriate recommendation that an adequate medical evaluation be performed to exclude other medical disorders, the authors take the reader through the principles of psychological assessment; the application of a symptom diary to identify predominant symptoms (as targets for improvement); and the assessment of comorbid psychiatric conditions, life stress, the social context of the symptoms, and the individual's social supports, beliefs and cognitions, and coping style. This section offers ample quotes, examples, and questions to bring the theoretical concepts into a here-and-now application. For example, questions are offered to help explore the ways in which the client's bowel symptoms fit into work, home life, and social relationships (e.g., "If there were no bowel disorder, how might your home life be different?").

The assessment of cognitions and coping style is particularly noteworthy. Relying on their extensive experience, the authors highlight the prominent issues that emerge with patients having IBS: bowel performance anxiety, control, social approval, sensitivity to social rules and norms, perfectionism, expression of anger, dealing with pain, self-efficacy, embarrassment/shame, and self-nurturance. The description of these themes, illustrated by case examples, serves as a primer for planning the direction of treatment.

The last four chapters provide the key features of treatment—a complete description of how to conduct a series of at least 12 sessions based on the key themes previously presented. Recommendations are offered on how to explain the basis for cognitive-behavioral treatment, how to address some of the "myths" that emerge (e.g., "If the pain is severe, there must be an organic cause."), and how to integrate the IBS-related themes into session-by-session exercises. The use of scripts and client–therapist dialogues is particularly valuable in demonstrating how the therapist can be effective in facilitating the client's learning.

As the field of medicine moves toward a more integrated,

biopsychosocial understanding of illness and disease and toward a relationship-centered plan of care, persons with IBS and other functional somatic syndromes are likely to benefit. This book paves the way toward that understanding and also provides the means to accomplish that goal.

Douglas A. Drossman, MD
Professor of Medicine and Psychiatry
Co-Director, UNC Center for Functional GI
  and Motility Disorders
University of North Carolina at Chapel Hill

Preface

The objective of this book is to describe a cognitive-behavioral treatment for irritable bowel syndrome (IBS). It is based on a theoretical and empirical understanding of cognitive-behavioral therapy and the biopsychosocial model of IBS. This cognitive-behavioral treatment approach for IBS has been adapted by our group in Toronto from an integration of work from the following cognitive-behavioral protocols: Beck and associates (Beck, 1976; Beck, Beck, Rush, Shaw, & Emery, 1979; Beck, Emery, & Greenberg, 1985) for the treatment of depressive and anxiety disorders; Turk, Meichenbaum, and Genest (1978) for chronic pain and stress management; Salkovskis (1989) for psychosomatic disorders; Lange and Jakubowski (1976) for assertiveness training; and Greenberger and Padesky (1995) for a cognitive therapy treatment manual for clients.

The impetus for the development of a cognitive-behavioral treatment for IBS follows the increasing recognition of the role played by attention allocation, personal appraisal style, and illness beliefs in chronic pain and psychosomatic disorders. In addition, the current efficacy of most medically based interventions in the treatment of IBS is not notably superior to placebo treatment, suggesting the need for new approaches to ameliorate the suffering of patients with IBS. The empirical literature has recently supported the use of cognitive-behavioral treatment for IBS (Toner et al., 1998).

In this volume, we outline the theoretical rationale for a cognitive-behavioral model in IBS, its physiological concomitants, the pathways leading to symptom expression, and the relevant targets for a cognitive-behavioral intervention strategy, along with a practical guide to treatment and data bearing on its efficacy. This book will appeal to clinicians working with clients with IBS, and will be of particular interest to mental health professionals, family physicians, and gastroenterologists, who frequently see patients with IBS in their practice. It should also appeal to researchers.

This book is divided into two parts. Part I focuses on a general overview of IBS and provides a rationale for the use of cognitive-behavioral treatment for IBS based on both theoretical and research perspectives. This section includes a critical review of cognitive-behavioral therapies for IBS and provides a model of cognitive-behavioral treatment. Part II focuses on the clinical application of cognitive-behavioral treatment with clients with IBS. This section provides the clinician with practical information concerning assessment issues as well as suggestions for initial and final sessions. We have provided suggestions for health professionals in this section. Common problems and troubleshooting are illustrated using possible scripts and case examples. However, these scripts are not intended to be used as a rule book but more as helpful guidelines. These scripts and case examples identify and highlight factors that may arise in working with clients with IBS relative to other clinical groups. Part II also contains an empirically tested cognitive-behavioral treatment protocol for clients with IBS using a group format. It is a menu-driven approach similar to that of *Mind over Mood* (Padesky & Greenberger, 1995) and includes suggested content areas for sessions based on the issues or themes that have been relevant for most clients with IBS in the research literature as well as in our clinical work. However, these issues are meant to serve as guidelines and should be tailored to the individual goals of clients in partnership with therapists. The individual issues/themes are presented in a specific order as a general guide for clinicians based on our empirical research. Contingent on the formulation of the presenting or emerging issues and goals, the order and inclusion of themes may be changed to fit the particular needs of a given individual or group.

Acknowledgments

We would like to acknowledge the many people who were important to us in the process of completing this work. First, we would like to extend our gratitude to the staff at The Guilford Press and especially recognize Seymour Weingarten, Barbara Watkins, and Anna Nelson for their endless patience, encouragement, and helpful feedback.

We would also like to recognize several students and staff who contributed helpful comments and/or technical assistance on earlier drafts of this book: Melissa Aiken, Donna Akman, Alisha Ali, Josee Casati, Meenu Chhabra, Kathy Downie, Ines DiGasbarro, Eileen Koyama, Dina Quattrochocchi, Sue Osborne, Noreen Stuckless, Taryn Tang, Claudia Van Duinen, Harriet Weaver, Betty Yu, and Therese Zarb.

We are grateful to the Ontario Mental Health Foundation for a grant that supported our research on cognitive-behavioral therapy for irritable bowel syndrome.

And, finally, we owe our deepest appreciation to the many individuals with irritable bowel syndrome who have shared their invaluable insights with us. We hope that this book will help to reduce the pain and stigma and increase the well-being of those who suffer from this disorder.

Contents

I

THEORETICAL AND RESEARCH PERSPECTIVES

1

Overview of Irritable Bowel Syndrome

Definition and Symptoms

Consensual criteria now exist (Drossman et al., 1994) to diagnose functional bowel disorders depending on the predominant symptoms: irritable bowel syndrome (IBS), functional constipation, functional diarrhea, and chronic functional abdominal pain.

Irritable bowel syndrome is the most common functional bowel disorder and is associated with continuous or recurrent symptoms for at least 3 months of the following:

1. Abdominal pain or discomfort, relieved with defecation or associated with a change in frequency or consistency of stool.
2. Two or more of the following, with at least one occurring on one-fourth of occasions or days:
   a. Altered stool frequency.
   b. Altered stool form (hard or loose/watery stool).
   c. Altered stool passage (straining or urgency, feeling of incomplete evacuation).
   d. Passage of mucus.
   e. Bloating or feeling of abdominal distension.

Epidemiology

IBS is very common in the North American adult population, with symptoms compatible with a diagnosis of IBS being reported in 9–22% of people (Drossman, Sandler, McKee, & Lovitz, 1982; Drossman et al., 1993; Sandler, 1990; Talley, Zinsmeister, Van Dyke, & Melton, 1991). However, the vast majority of those who have IBS symptoms do not seek medical attention for those concerns (Whitehead, Bosmaijian, Zonderman, Costa, & Schuster, 1988). The subgroup that seeks medical consultation accounts for 12% of primary care and 28% of gastroenterological practice in Western societies (Drossman et al., 1997). This disorder leads to over 2 million prescriptions per year in the United States (Sandler, 1990) and is associated with unnecessary and often harmful tests, procedures, and surgeries (Burns, 1986; Thompson, Dotevall, Drossman, Heaton, & Kruis, 1989). Whitehead et al. (1990) found that 21% of patients with IBS in their sample had undergone hysterectomies for treatment of their gastrointestinal symptoms. This is significantly higher than the national U.S. average of 5.5%. In addition to the cost to the health care system, the general economic impact of IBS is considerable. IBS has been ranked as the second most common cause of industrial absenteeism due to illness (Young, Alpers, Norland, & Woodruff, 1976).

Studies examining the prevalence of IBS symptoms show that within the nonpatient population, the ratio of female to male sufferers is two to one. Within the patient population that seeks consultation with primary care physicians, females outnumber males by three to one. In tertiary care settings, female patients are four or five times more prevalent than male patients. Given that the majority of patients with IBS are women, clearly, it must be regarded as a women's health issue. As reviewed by Toner and Akman (1999), most studies on IBS use only women in their samples, and of those studies that include men, few test for sex differences. Even when sex differences are explored, due to small sample sizes, investigators often qualify their findings, making it difficult to generalize results. When differences between the sexes are reported, they are often descriptive, with no reference to whether any of the findings have reached statistical significance. Studies that include both men and women in their sample and examine for sex differences have focused their investigation in the areas of frequency of physician visits, physical symptomatology, psychological symptomatology, and abuse histories. A review of this literature shows that in tests for statistical significance, few consistent sex differences are found. Accordingly, to date, most of our information about IBS has been drawn from women participants. Chapter 3 details some of the emerging themes that have been found in women presenting with IBS. Future studies should include more male clients with IBS in their samples, for until we know more about males who seek treatment for IBS, we will be unable to make any definitive statements about similarities or differences in themes between the sexes.

Predisposing, Precipitating, and Perpetuating Factors

Several predisposing, precipitating, and perpetuating factors of IBS have been identified as contributing to the expression and maintenance of IBS symptoms. To date, no physiological or psychosocial markers have been identified. As summarized by Drossman (1996), IBS is best conceptualized using a biopsychosocial framework. Symptoms may be generated from physiological disturbances (enhanced motility and visceral sensation) that are closely connected to central nervous system activity (via the central nervous system–enteric nervous system axis). The clinical expression of these symptoms (e.g., a person's illness behavior, the decision to take medication or seek health care) is strongly influenced by psychosocial factors. For this reason, the high frequency of psychosocial distress (e.g., high life stress, psychiatric diagnoses, sexual abuse history) in the absence of modulating factors (e.g., social support, coping strategies) reported among patients with IBS may in part relate to their self-selection into referral practices. Studies have revealed that patients with IBS who do not seek health care do not differ significantly from healthy controls on several psychological parameters (Drossman et al., 1988; Whitehead et al., 1988; Drossman et al., 1990). Recently, there has been much attention directed to brain–gut interactions as a useful explanatory model for IBS.

Brain–Gut Interactions

As summarized by Drossman et al. (1999), a unifying hypothesis to explain the functional gastrointestinal disorders in general, and IBS in particular, is that they result from dysregulation of "brain–gut" neuroenteric systems, which is a dysregulation of central nervous system–neuroenteric system pathways rather than a disease of any of these structures. For a less technical description of brain–gut interaction, readers are referred to Chapter 5. It is no longer rational to try to determine whether psychological or physiological factors cause pain or other bowel symptoms. Both are operative, and the task is to determine the degree to which each contributes and is remediable. When compared to healthy subjects, patients with functional gastrointestinal disorders have increased motor reactivity to various stressors, including balloon distension, food, various peptides, and physical and psychological stressors. Furthermore, patients with IBS have decreased thresholds for gut pain in response to balloon distension and other stimuli (visceral hypersensitivity). The role of the central nervous system in modulating motility is supported by evidence that (1) the motility disturbances in IBS disappear during sleep; (2) patients with IBS have a different electroencephalographic sleep pattern than healthy subjects; (3) migrating motor complex (MMC) frequency decreases and propagating velocity increases progressively with alertness and arousal; and (4) experimental stressors appear to have linked effects leading to simultaneous increases in electroencephalographic beta power activity and colonic motility that are significantly greater in patients with IBS.

The role of the central nervous system in modulating visceral perception is supported by recent studies using positron emission tomography, which differentiates patients with IBS from a nonclinical comparison group based on regional cerebral perfusion. When evaluating the central nervous system response to rectal distension, or even the anticipation of rectal distension, patients with IBS, compared to controls, fail to activate the anterior cingulate cortex, an area of the limbic system associated with active opiate binding, but do activate the prefrontal cortex, an area associated with hypervigilance and anxiety. Therefore, patients with IBS may fail to use central nervous system down-regulating mechanisms in response to incoming or anticipated visceral pain. Instead, they may activate an area of the brain that amplifies pain perception. Cognitive-behavioral techniques may help increase activation in the anterior cingulate cortex and parts of the brain that amplify pain, reduce activation, and thus reduce pain perception.

As reviewed by Drossman et al. (1999), the varied influence of environmental stress, thoughts, and emotions on gut function effected through neurotransmitter release or receptor activity may explain the remarkable variation in symptoms of patients having these disorders. For example, patients with IBS can have both constipation and diarrhea, or disturbed motility without pain, or even pain without dysmotility ("altered perception of normal function"). It also helps explain how psychosocial trauma (e.g., physical, emotional, or sexual abuse history) or unhelpful coping style (e.g., "catastrophizing") profoundly affect symptom severity, daily function, and health outcome. This is where psychosocial factors in general and cognitive-behavioral perspectives in particular can play a central role in both our understanding and treatment of IBS. We briefly review psychosocial factors before discussing treatment issues.

Psychosocial Factors

Research has repeatedly demonstrated a significant psychological component in patients who seek specialized medical consultation for IBS. In particular, numerous studies have demonstrated a high prevalence of psychiatric illness (50–100%) in patients with IBS (MacDonald & Bouchier, 1980; Colgan, Creed, & Klass, 1988; Corney & Stanton, 1990; Craig & Brown, 1984; Ford, Miller, Eastwood, & Eastwood, 1987; Toner, Garfinkel, Jeejeebhoy, Scher, et al., 1990; Blanchard, Scharff, Schwartz, Suls, & Barlow, 1990). There is much current debate about the relationship between IBS and psychiatric disorders (i.e., that of a cause, consequence, or co-occurrence).

In addition to the high frequency of psychiatric illness, especially depression and anxiety disorders, various psychological symptoms, characteristics, and behaviors have been reported in patients. Severe life stress has been found immediately before the onset of functional bowel disorders (Creed, Craig, & Farmer, 1988). For many patients, social stress plays an important part in explaining exacerbation of symptoms and treatment seeking. Like patients with other medical disorders, patients with IBS have higher psychosocial distress scores than people without health problems or a nonclinical population with similar gastrointestinal complaints (Drossman et al., 1997). However, there is no personality profile unique to IBS. Patients with IBS who seek health care (Drossman et al., 1988; Whitehead et al., 1988), particularly at specialty clinics, have more severe medical symptoms and more anxiety, depression (Drossman et al., 1988; Heaton et al., 1992; Talley, Boyce, & Jones, 1997), and health anxiety (Drossman et al., 1988), and they are less likely to see a link between stress and their IBS symptoms (Toner, 1994; Thompson, Heaton, Smyth, & Smyth, 1996). Patients with IBS commonly believe that their bowel symptoms indicate serious gut disease/cancer, and they attend selectively to abdominal sensations and seek out information that is consistent with such beliefs (Toner et al., 1998b). Patients with IBS report many nongastrointestinal symptoms (Chabbra, Toner, Ali, & Stuckless, 1999). They make two to three times more visits to physicians for nongastrointestinal problems (Drossman et al., 1993) and report missing an average of 13.4 days from work or usual activities due to illness compared to 4.9 days for the whole sample (Drossman et al., 1993; Kellow, Gill, & Wingate, 1990). The implication of these findings is that patients with IBS may benefit from psychological interventions, which, in addition to reducing gastrointestinal symptoms, may also reduce subjective distress and enable them to cope with this chronic disorder. While both physiological and psychosocial factors have been identified as important in the treatment of IBS, to date, intervention has mainly focused on medications and dietary fiber. While a comprehensive review of physiological interventions is beyond the scope of this book, the reader is referred to Drossman et al. (1999) for a review.

Psychological Interventions

The importance of psychological factors in patients who seek repeated specialized consultation for IBS has been well documented in the literature (Drossman et al., 1995). However, there have been surprisingly few controlled studies investigating psychological treatments for patients with IBS. One of the most challenging problems in reviewing the literature on psychological interventions for IBS is that most of the controlled studies have used multicomponent treatment packages that comprise various combinations of cognitive-behavioral, relaxation, psychodynamic, and biofeedback approaches. Consequently, the efficacy of a specific theoretical approach is difficult to assess. Moreover, investigators in general do not adequately describe their therapeutic techniques and procedures. A summary of the various multicomponent and individual treatment approaches to IBS are shown in Tables 1.1 and 1.2. Before discussing interventions that have substantive cognitive-behavioral components in their treatment packages (Table 1.2), we briefly review psychological interventions, including psychodynamic therapy, hypnosis, and relaxation interventions of various combinations in multicomponent treatment packages (Table 1.1).

In a study focusing on short-term psychodynamic therapy, Guthrie, Creed, Dawson, and Tomenson (1991) used progressive

TABLE 1.1. Psychological Interventions That Did Not Use Cognitive-Behavioral Therapy

Study	Psychodynamic	Relaxation	Hypnosis
Svedlund (1983)	×		
Guthrie, Creed, Dawson, & Tomenson (1991)	×	×	
Voirol & Hipolito (1987)		×	
Blanchard, Greene, Scharff, & Schwarz-McMorris (1993)		×	
Whorwell, Prior, & Faragher (1984)			×
Whorwell, Prior, & Colgan (1987)			×
Harvey, Hinton, & Gunary (1989)			×

TABLE 1.2. Interventions That Used Cognitive-Behavioral Therapy

	Cognitive-behavioral	Relaxation	Biofeedback	Education	Psycho-dynamic
Arn, Theorell, Uvnas-Moberg, & Jonsson (1989)	×	×			×
Lynch & Zamble (1989)	×	×			
Corney, Stanton, Newell, Clare, & Fairclough (1991)	×				
Bennett & Wilkinson (1985)	×	×		×	
Shaw et al. (1991)	×	×			
Rumsey (1991)	×	×		×	
Blanchard et al. (1992)	×	×	×	×	
Neff & Blanchard (1987)	×	×	×	×	
Greene & Blanchard (1994)	×				
Payne & Blanchard (1995)	×				
Vollmer & Blanchard (1998)	×				
Van Dulmen, Fennis, & Bleijenberg (1996)	×	×			
Toner et al. (1998b)	×	×			

muscle relaxation training as an adjunct to exploratory psychotherapy and found that combined treatment was superior to medical management alone. Specifically, they found that clients with IBS in the psychotherapy condition had significant improvement on ratings of diarrhea and abdominal pain, and this was associated with reductions in depression, anxiety, and patient visits.

Arn, Theorell, Uvnas-Moberg, and Jonsson (1989) used an unspecified form of relaxation training as an adjunct to psychodrama and found that this combined treatment was more effective than standard medical therapy for reducing anxiety, but it was not more effective for reducing gastrointestinal symptoms. A low participation rate (21%) mars the interpretation of this study.

Svedlund (1983) compared psychodynamic therapy to continuation of routine medical care and found that with regard to bowel dysfunction and abdominal pain, the psychotherapy group improved more than controls. The difference became more pronounced 1 year later, when the psychotherapy group showed further improvement on measures of anxiety and depression, in addition to gastrointestinal symptoms, compared with the control group.

Voirol and Hipolito (1987) compared 6 months of treatment with conventional medical therapy to 6 months of treatment with relaxation exercises and reported that the relaxation group showed significantly fewer pain episodes and visits to medical clinics 40 months after treatment.

Blanchard, Greene, Scharff, and Schwarz-McMorris (1993) reported a comparison of a group undergoing relaxation training alone to a symptom-monitoring control group. The relaxation group showed significantly more reduction in gastrointestinal symptoms than the control group. One-half of the relaxation group improved by at least 50%, a figure comparable to previous reports with Blanchard's multicomponent treatment.

Whorwell, Prior, and Faragher (1984) randomized 30 subjects to receive either hypnosis or a control treatment. Clients were instructed to place a hand on their abdomen and feel a sense of warmth, and relate this to asserting control over gut function. They were also instructed to use visual imagery (e.g., a river flowing) to decrease gastrointestinal contractions. The control treatment in this study consisted of discussions of symptoms and the possible contribution of emotional problems and stress to IBS, plus a placebo tablet. The hypnotherapy group showed significantly greater reductions in bowel symptoms and improvement in the sense of well-being. Subsequently, Whorwell, Prior, and Colgan (1987) reported follow-up data showing that these 15 subjects had maintained their treatment gains at 18 months. In follow-up reports, which were not controlled studies, Whorwell and colleagues described the treatment of additional clients (more than 200) with hypnosis and reported that their overall success rate was 85% (Whorwell et al., 1987). Age greater than

50 years and the presence of high levels of anxiety were predictors of poorer outcomes with hypnotherapy.

Harvey, Hinton, Gunary, and Barry (1989) replicated the work of Whorwell and compared hypnotherapy in groups to individual hypnotherapy. Twenty of 33 clients benefited, and those treated in groups were as likely to improve as those treated individually. Like Whorwell, these researchers found that symptoms of psychological distress predicted a poorer response to hypnosis.

Review of Cognitive-Behavioral Therapies

Within the last decade, in addition to the intervention by our group in Toronto, there have been several controlled studies involving cognitive and/or behavioral therapy packages. While these studies are promising in that they support cognitive-behavioral principles in the treatment of IBS, they all suffer from substantial methodological flaws that limit the interpretation of their findings. Moreover, although the vast majority of clients in these studies were women, the variable of gender was not addressed as either a conceptual or treatment issue in these reports.

A study by Bennett and Wilkinson (1985) compared an 8-week psychological treatment package (i.e., stress management training, cognitive therapy, and contingency management) and a medical treatment consisting of a daily drug regimen (Motival, Mebererine, Fybosel). Anxiety levels were reduced in the psychological, but not the medical, intervention. IBS symptoms and associated behaviors (e.g., restriction of activity, fatigue, verbal complaints of pain or discomfort) were reduced in both groups. This study, however, suffers from several methodological shortcomings: It does not adequately describe or monitor therapeutic techniques; follow-up data were not provided; global ratings that overestimate change (Neff & Blanchard, 1987) were used; and there was no control for possible attention placebo effects, as the medical controls were only seen monthly for 15-minute consultations.

Shaw et al. (1991) combined cognitive-behavioral therapy strategies, relaxation techniques, and educational components in their stress management program for IBS. This program appeared to be more effective in reducing the frequency and intensity of symptoms compared to "conventional" therapy, which included Colpermin. Benefits were maintained at 12-month follow-up.

Rumsey (1991) likewise combined progressive muscle relaxation training with education and cognitive-behavioral therapy for stress management. His clients were treated in small groups and were compared to clients treated with anticholinergic medications, psychotropics, and bulking agents; the behavior therapy group did not receive drugs. At the end of treatment, gastrointestinal symptoms had declined to a similar extent in the two groups, but the cognitive-behavioral therapy group showed greater reduction in depression and anxiety. At 6-month follow-up, the cognitive-behavioral group had fewer gastrointestinal symptoms than the pharmacologically treated group.

Lynch and Zamble (1989) also reported on a multicomponent method, which they called a behavioral treatment package. Although the treatment package was similar to that of Blanchard's group, it replaced thermal biofeedback with assertiveness training. The behavioral group improved significantly more than a wait-list control group in both IBS symptoms and measures of mood and self-perceptions. Therapeutic gains were maintained over a 5-month follow-up period. Interpretation of findings was limited by the following: While approximately 80 persons were scheduled to receive treatment, only 30 agreed to participate, limiting the generalizability of the findings; no active placebo control group was included to control for the effects of being in therapy; no information was provided on the number and experience level of the therapists; and no adherence-to-protocol ratings were taken.

Neff and Blanchard (1987) compared a multicomponent treatment program (educational information, progressive relaxation therapy, thermal biofeedback treatment, coping skills) to a symptom-monitoring control condition. Treatment was effective in reducing gastrointestinal symptoms (as measured by a daily diary) in 6 out of 10 clients with IBS in the active treatment group, while individuals in the symptom-monitoring condition showed little change. The symptom-monitoring group was then offered treatment and more than half of this group improved. Since the control group was offered treatment during follow-up, this study was limited by its absence of a follow-up assessment. In a 4-year follow-up report, the majority of clients treated maintained symptom reduction. In addition, the following four weaknesses limited interpretation of this psychological intervention: (1) All treatments were conducted by the same therapist, so that the effects could be due to the therapist and not the therapy per se; (2) the study did not control for therapist attention or the effects of "being in treatment"; (3) it is not possible to identify which parts of this multicomponent program were responsible for outcome; (4) no adherence to treatment protocol ratings were taken.

In an extension of their earlier work, Blanchard's group (Blanchard et al., 1992) improved their methodology by comparing the active multicomponent treatment package with an attention placebo control group in addition to the wait-list control group. Results indicated that the active multicomponent group treatment package did not show any significant gains over the placebo group. However, since this multicomponent package invested a substantial percentage of time on thermal biofeedback in addition to cognitive components, it is not possible to determine which components were effective. Moreover, inexperienced therapists (i.e., students) were used in this study.

Blanchard's group recently addressed many of these methodological issues in a well-controlled cognitive therapy intervention for clients with IBS. The first study found greater gastrointestinal symptom reduction for clients with IBS randomly assigned to cognitive therapy than for those in the symptom-monitoring control group (Greene & Blanchard, 1994). The second study tested a cognitive therapy group against a self-help support group and found significant improvement in IBS symptoms, depression, and anxiety in the cognitive therapy group (Payne & Blanchard, 1995). The third study (Vollmer & Blanchard, 1998) showed improvement on gastrointestinal symptoms in both individual and group cognitive therapy compared with a symptom-monitoring group. Results for all three studies were upheld at 3-month follow-up assessment. Finally, Van Dulmen et al. (1996) found improvement in abdominal pain, coping strategies, and avoidance behavior in their cognitive-behavioral therapy group relative to a wait-list control group. Long-term improvement was maintained.

While these previous studies demonstrate the effectiveness of cognitive-behavioral therapy, we (Toner et al.,1998b) recently completed a study that improved upon them by (1) using a detailed session-by-session manual to enable experimental and control groups to maintain consistency; (2) employing experienced cognitive-behavioral therapists to conduct the groups; (3) audiotaping all sessions and randomly selecting tapes to check for adherence to protocol; (4) measuring effect using a daily diary of bowel symptoms rather than a global self-report; (5) including 6-month follow-up assessment; and (6) comparing cognitive-behavioral and education–attention placebo conditions against usual medical treatment. We next describe our treatment study including the basic design, treatment interventions, and preliminary findings.

Overview of Our Treatment Study

Basic Design

The sample consisted of a total of 101 individuals ages 18–65 who received a diagnosis of IBS. The sample was randomly assigned to one of the following three conditions: (1) a cognitive-behavioral group treatment; (2) a psychoeducational group treatment; (3) conventional medical treatment. All dependent measures were administered at preintervention, postintervention, and 6-month follow-up.

Treatment Intervention

COGNITIVE-BEHAVIORAL GROUP

The treatment protocol used by our group in Toronto is derived from work by Shaw (1979), Hollon and Shaw (1979), Covi, Roth, and Lipman (1982), and Covi and Lipman (1987). It consists of a closed-ended group (i.e., all group members start and finish treatment at the same time). The group includes 12 weekly, 90-

minute sessions and has a membership of 6 clients with one therapist. While we included 6 clients over 12 group sessions in our treatment protocol, we suggest that the size of the group and number of sessions could range from 4 to 8 clients over 10 to 20 sessions.

At each of the 12 group sessions, a predetermined agenda as well as individual agenda items were chosen by each group member for that session. The agenda is described in detail in Chapter 5.

One individual treatment session is conducted prior to the beginning of the first group session (i.e., initial session), its purpose being to begin discussing the theoretical and therapeutic rationale for cognitive-behavioral therapy with clients. In particular, the cognitive-behavioral model is used to highlight how certain cognitions and underlying beliefs may lead to increased attention to bodily sensations, increased arousal, and heightened sensitivity to pain and other IBS symptoms. The model takes into account how IBS symptoms may become perpetuated by an interplay among biological, psychological, and social factors. A second purpose of the individual session is to establish initial rapport with the client and identify treatment goals. A second individual session is conducted following the sixth group session. The purpose of this session is to clarify any issues regarding the group and to review the individual's progress in the group.

It should be noted that progressive relaxation is not part of the treatment protocol for the cognitive group therapy as outlined by the aforementioned authors. It was added as a behavioral component of cognitive-behavioral therapy based on our rationale described earlier. Also, relaxation has proven useful in the treatment of anxiety disorders (Beck et al., 1985).

PSYCHOEDUCATIONAL GROUP

The psychoeducational group was identical to the cognitive-behavioral group in terms of length and frequency of sessions (i.e., individual and group) and group membership. It follows a modified protocol described by Buchanan (1978) for chronic physically ill patients. This protocol was adapted by Wise, Cooper, and Ahmed (1982) for clients with IBS. Buchanan describes his protocol as a two-phase program. The earlier sessions (Phase 1) were aimed at client education about their disorder. Each meeting began in a highly structured and didactic manner using audiovisual aids and reading materials. A discussion period followed in which members were encouraged to comment on the information presented. The later sessions had a psychological orientation directed at supportive therapy. In the earlier sessions (Phase 1) of our psychoeducational group, the anatomy and pathophysiology of IBS were presented. In addition, dietary factors and life events that may aggravate the condition were described. Phase 2 consisted of supportive therapy in which members were encouraged to discuss their difficulties.

CONVENTIONAL MEDICAL GROUP

Patients randomly assigned to this condition received the usual medical treatment that was given by the referring gastroenterologist to patients with IBS. Contingent on the clinical presentation of a given individual, this could range from no treatment to any combination of physiological interventions. The type of intervention and number (and duration) of medical contacts were monitored over the course of the study.

In order to ensure that all participants perceived the rationale for their group treatment to be equally credible, we asked participants in the cognitive-behavioral and psychoeducational groups to provide ratings on this dimension using the Scale for Treatment Rationale Credibility Rating (Borkovec & Nau, 1972). It should be noted that unless contraindicated, medical intervention for patients in both groups was kept to a minimum. If a physiological agent was judged by the gastroenterologist to be clinically indicated for cognitive-behavioral and psychoeducational groups, this information was recorded and taken into consideration in the data analysis.

The following initial findings were reported for pre- and postassessment times for 101 patients (Toner et al., 1998b).

1. *Beck Depression Inventory.* As predicted, on scores for the Beck Depression Inventory, a significant group × time interaction was found at time 1 versus time 2, $F(2,97) = 8.01$; $p < .001$. Analysis of simple effects showed that the cognitive-behavioral therapy group improved significantly on this measure, $t(97) = 2.24$; $p < .05$, while the medical control group showed an increase in depression scores, $t(97) = 2.85$; $p < .01$, and the psychoeducational group showed no significant change on this measure. These findings indicate that clients in the cognitive-behavioral therapy group improved more significantly on depression scores than did clients in either the psychoeducational group or the conventional medical group.

2. *Marlowe–Crowne Social Desirability Scale.* As predicted, there was a significant group × time interaction found on the Marlowe–Crowne Social Desirability Scale (Crowne & Marlowe, 1960), $F(2,96) = 5.02$; $p < .01$. Analysis of simple effects showed a decrease in social desirability in the cognitive-behavioral therapy group, $t(96) = 2.40$; $p < .02$. This is noteworthy, since our cognitive-behavioral therapy model suggests that social desirability (i.e., heightened need to present oneself in a favorable light) is a central cognition in clients with IBS. This study is the first to demonstrate that cognitive-behavioral therapy can significantly reduce need for social desirability in clients with IBS. Neither the psychoeducational nor the medical control groups showed a significant change on this measure.

3. *Gastrointestinal Symptoms Diary.* Scores reported on the Gastrointestinal Symptoms Diary were generally low at pretest assessments. Thus, analyses controlling for "floor effects" were performed on these data. This was accomplished by including clients who had experienced at least two gastrointestinal symptoms per week over the course of the 2-week baseline period. As predicted, after controlling for floor effects, a significant group × time interaction, $F(1,34) = 5.55$; $p < .05$, on severity of bloating was found. Simple effects showed a significant decrease in the cognitive-behavioral therapy group as compared to the medical control group, $t(34) = 2.23$; $p < .01$, demonstrating that the cognitive-behavioral therapy group improved significantly more than the medical control group on bloating. We did not find significant group × time interactions on the symptoms of diarrhea, constipa-

tion, pain, and tenderness, possibly due to the small numbers of clients involved in these analyses after controlling for floor effects. We conducted repeated measures analyses on these four symptoms and found that the cognitive-behavioral therapy group reported significant improvement from time 1 to time 2 on diarrhea, $t(11) = 2.23; p < .05$, constipation, $t(15) = 2.27; p < .02$, pain, $t(18) = 3.88; p < .001$, and tenderness, $t(16) = 2.42; p < .05$. As expected, the psychoeducational and medical control groups did not show any significant changes in diarrhea, constipation, pain, and tenderness.

4. *Therapy Efficacy Questionnaire.* The Therapy Efficacy Questionnaire is a 12-item questionnaire developed by our group (Toner et al., 1998b) to assess clients' perceptions of the effectiveness or usefulness of the therapy. This questionnaire has shown internal consistency, with a reliability coefficient of .84. As predicted, a *t*-test using the total scores on this measure revealed that at post assessment, subjects in the cognitive-behavioral group reported significantly higher therapy efficacy scores than did psychoeducational group subjects, $t(48) = 4.37; p < .01$. The following items significantly differed between groups, with the cognitive-behavioral group scoring significantly higher than the psychoeducational group on each item:

"I have incorporated the information learned in the group into my daily activities." $(t = 2.24; p < .05)$

"I am engaging in activities that I would not have been able to do prior to participating in the group." $(t = 2.96; p < .01)$

"I am better able to cope with my symptoms as a result of participating in the group." $(t = 2.80; p < .01)$

"Participation in the group has helped me to cope better in other areas of my life." $(t = 3.01; p < .01)$

"My IBS symptoms have improved as a result of participating in the group." $(t = 3.47; p < .01)$

"I would recommend this group to other people with IBS." $(t = 2.57; p < .02)$

"My level of confidence has increased as a result of participating in the group." $(t = 2.31; p < .05)$

"I found the group to be more helpful than I had expected." $(t = 4.78; p < .01)$

It should be noted that every individual who attended the cognitive-behavioral treatment group positively endorsed the item "I would recommend this group to other people with IBS." Based on the Credibility Scale adapted from Borkovec and Nau (1972), we also found that there were no differences in initial expectations between individuals in the cognitive-behavioral group and the psychoeducational group.

2

Cognitive-Behavioral Treatment for IBS

Cognitive-Behavioral Model for IBS

The cognitive-behavioral model presented here was adapted from a model developed by Sharpe, Peveler, and Mayou (1992) for functional somatic syndromes. Other investigators have used similar models to describe various psychiatric and psychological conditions (Barsky, Geringer, & Wool, 1988; Beck et al., 1985; Hawton et al., 1989; Mayou, 1989; Salkovskis & Warwick, 1986; Warwick & Salkovskis, 1990). Central to the cognitive-behavioral model is the way the person thinks about his/her bowel symptoms. If the bowel symptoms are attributed to disease or organic causes, then the person may seek out medical consultation for a medical explanation of his/her difficulties. A large percentage of people who consult a physician are reassured by the negative findings. A small percentage of patients (or their physicians) are not reassured and may be referred to a specialist for more extensive investigations. Some patients still may feel that something has been missed or overlooked by the specialist and seek out other gastrointestinal specialists or consult various nonmedical therapists in the persistent search for more extensive investigation.

According to a cognitive-behavioral model, IBS symptoms and distress are perpetuated by an interaction between psychological, social, and physiological factors. Cognitions such as "There must be a medical explanation for this pain" lead to certain behaviors (e.g., further medical consultations), increased attention, and hypervigilance of bodily sensations, increased anxiety, and arousal that may lead to a heightened sensitivity to pain. During this process, sensations become amplified and are experienced as more noxious and intense, which may then lead to further thoughts that something must have been overlooked, and to further physiological arousal and self-scrutiny that amplifies other bodily sensations. These new sensations may be taken as confirmatory evidence of a physical cause. Independent of the predisposing factors related to the symptoms, cognitions about the illness and the associated anxiety serve to maintain and amplify the symptoms. Using a simple example such as a "mosquito bite" serves to highlight the influence of selective attention on heightened sensations (e.g., the more you focus on the bite, the more it itches. The more it itches, the more you scratch it. The more you scratch it, the redder, sorer, and itchier it is, and so on).

Consistent with an information-processing model, people selectively attend to those cognitions and perceptions that confirm their explanatory hypotheses while selectively ignoring information or sensory input that is inconsistent with their beliefs (Barsky et al., 1988). Accordingly, other possible contributing factors such as life stressors, psychological distress, overwork, interpersonal conflict, or loss may be minimized or selected out of individuals' conceptualization of their IBS symptoms. There is some empirical support for this model in the work of Drossman and colleagues (1988), who found that individuals with IBS who sought out specialized consultation for their symptoms (i.e., patients with IBS) were significantly more likely to minimize psychological and stress-related factors in their lives relative to a comparison group of individuals with IBS who did not consult specialists for their symptoms (i.e., IBS nonpatients). In addition, Levy, Cain, Jarriett, and Heitkemper (1997) found that patients with IBS were less likely to report an association between IBS symptoms and stressors relative to IBS nonpatients.

In the persistent search for organic causes, both patient and doctor become frustrated and the doctor–patient relationship is compromised. This can lead to various scenarios that serve further to heighten patients' (and doctors') distress and fuel the vicious circle of perpetuating factors. Since the patient is hypervigilant to any hint that medical specialists, friends, family, employer, or society are not taking his/her symptoms seriously, he/she will try "harder" or become even more determined to find the medical cause for their very real pain and physical suffering. Patients with IBS, who have high moral standards and heightened need for approval (Toner, Koyamia, Garfinkel, Jeejeebhoy, & DiGasbarro, 1992), are especially hypervigilant to the negative stigma and moral connotations associated with any psychological explanation of their symptoms.

Our group has reported findings that confirm clinical descriptions of the need for clients with IBS to present themselves in a socially desirable manner. Specifically, we found that clients with IBS had a significantly higher L-Score than nonclinical controls on the Eysenck Personality Inventory, indicating a response style that aims to present oneself in a favorable light by endorsing socially approved items (Toner, Garfinkel, & Jeejeebhoy, 1990). This finding is supported in our data analysis on the Marlowe–Crowne Social Desirability Scale in which clients with IBS have significantly higher scores than age-matched psychiatric outpatients with major depression and nonclinical control groups (Toner et al., 1992). In addition, we found that on a test of self-schema (i.e., knowledge of self stored in memory), clients with IBS with major depression recall more nondepressed words describing self compared to a psychiatric outpatient group with major depression (Toner, Garfinkel, Jeejeebhoy, Scher, et al., 1990). In other words, clients with IBS with major depression do not view themselves as depressed.

On the basis of these findings, together with earlier descriptions, we propose a conceptual model based on the notion that some clients with IBS may adopt a self-schema characterized by social desirability. Such a model may contribute to our understanding of why individuals with similar psychological symptoms (e.g., depression, anxiety) present to either mental health professionals or gastroenterologists because they, respectively, identify their problems as psychological or organic in nature (Toner et al., 1992). Moreover, we postulate that this heightened need for social approval is reinforced in our Western society in general, and in medicine in particular, by the continued stigma associated with psychologically based explanations for somatically based symptoms (Kirmayer & Robbins, 1991).

This heightened arousal and attention leads to further amplification of symptoms and a filtering out of information that is incompatible with the client's explanatory model of his/her IBS. Consequently, IBS symptoms become intensified and perpetuated by the cognitions, forming a vicious circle. According to Kirmayer and Robbins (1991), clients with functional somatic syndromes may also experience added worry, self-doubt, and public scrutiny due to the ambiguity and "unreality" of their illness. This negation of their experience may heighten certain forms of illness behavior such as the adamant rejection of psychological causation in an effort to obtain medical and social validation for their suffering. This pattern of illness behavior is an interaction among predisposing factors that is accentuated and perpetuated by the medical system and society.

We find that clients who feel that their IBS symptoms are being taken seriously and are helped through cognitive and behavioral techniques are more willing to accept treatment of any associated psychosocial problems and to alter unhelpful illness behaviors. In our cognitive-behavioral group work with clients with IBS, unhelpful cognitions may have to do with IBS symptoms or other issues (e.g., relationships, achievements) and are usually expressed in extreme, all-or-nothing terms (e.g., I must get home when I begin to have bowel symptoms; I must do my absolute best at everything).

Key Characteristics of Cognitive-Behavioral Treatment

Cognitive-behavioral treatment consists of a wide range of strategies and procedures designed to bring about alterations in clients' perceptions of their situation and thus their ability to control their condition. The rationale for cognitive-behavioral strategies assumes that individuals can learn new ways of thinking and behaving through personal experience and practice.

In this section, we consider some key characteristics of cognitive-behavioral treatment. This is followed by a discussion of behavioral and cognitive intervention strategies.

Collaborative Empiricism

Cognitive-behavioral treatment distinguishes itself from many other psychotherapeutic approaches in its insistence upon "collaborative empiricism" as the *modus operandi*. This term highlights two important features of cognitive-behavioral treatment. First, cognitive-behavioral therapists seek to establish collaborative working alliances with clients. Therapists and clients work together to identify and track target problems, to generate strategies for change, and to execute and evaluate these strategies. Second, therapists encourage clients to view their thoughts as scientific hypotheses that can be tested empirically. As such, cognitive change is presumed to occur when clients, in collaboration with their therapists, repeatedly generate opportunities to compare and contrast their thoughts (expectations, assumptions, beliefs, etc.) with actual outcomes. This "evidence gathering" approach contrasts with other cognitively oriented therapies, notably rational–emotive therapy (Ellis & Dryden, 1987), which emphasizes the role of logical disputation and persuasion in promoting cognitive change. It can also be compared to psychodynamic treatments, in which the nature of the therapeutic relationship is interpretive rather than collaborative.

Use of Questions

A foundational therapeutic skill in cognitive-behavioral treatment relates to use of questioning. Beck et al. (1979) enumerated a number of important therapeutic functions served by a question-asking orientation. Framing verbalizations in the form of questions may facilitate translating clients' personal axioms into tentative hypotheses. This sets the stage for a consideration of self-generated alternatives and subsequent experimentation. In addition, the use of questioning (rather than indoctrination or overly aggressive disputation) can serve to promote a collaborative, respectful therapeutic alliance in which therapists may help clients to focus their concerns, explore the evidence for their beliefs, identify the criteria for their evaluations, and examine the consequences of their actions.

Here-and-Now Focus

Cognitive-behavioral treatment has, as one goal, the interruption of the vicious cycle of cognition, mood, and behavior that is associated with IBS. As such, it maintains a predominantly here-and-now focus. This stance does not imply a view of historical material as irrelevant or unimportant. Indeed, there is convergent evidence that unhelpful attitudes and beliefs may arise from negative early experience (Kovacs & Beck, 1978; for a review, see Brewin, Andrews, & Gotlib, 1993). Furthermore, and as we will point out later, exploring the developmental antecedents of unhelpful thinking patterns represents one approach to promoting schematic change. However, in cognitive-behavioral treatment, emphasis is placed on identifying and addressing the cognitive components that play a role in maintaining and amplifying symptoms. Consequently, clients' current concerns generally constitute the "raw material" for therapeutic attention. In this regard, it should be noted that events transpiring within the therapy session itself (e.g., the client's thoughts or feelings about the therapist, occurring quite literally in the here and now) may constitute a highly relevant clinical focus (for a detailed discussion of interpersonal process in cognitive-behavioral treatment, see Safran & Segal, 1990).

Use of Self-Help Assignments

In cognitive-behavioral treatment, therapists and clients typically work together to generate assignments that clients can carry out between sessions. In early sessions, assignments may involve the maintenance of daily records of mood, behavior, and/or unhelpful thoughts. Alternatively, and in keeping with the cognitive-behavioral emphasis on empiricism, assignments outside of the sessions may take the form of behavioral experiments designed to test empirical support for clients' thoughts, beliefs, or assumptions. In circumstances where a new behavioral skill is being developed (e.g., assertiveness), assignments may involve the strategic, real-life application of these skills. Whatever their form, self-help assignments constitute an integral component of treatment. Indeed, the tendency to complete assignments has been linked to superior therapeutic response (Neimeyer & Feixas, 1990). Furthermore, there is also evidence to suggest that those therapists who regularly take up and review assignments obtain better clinical outcomes than those who fail to do so (Burns & Nolen-Hoeksema, 1991; Williams, 1992).

Short-Term Orientation

Finally, cognitive-behavioral treatment is generally conducted on a short-term basis. Standard treatment protocols (e.g., Beck et al., 1979) recommend up to 20 sessions. The short-term focus establishes clear temporal parameters for therapy that can facilitate the motivation of both client and therapist to maintain a problem-centered orientation. In addition, it increases the importance of a clear formulation on the part of the therapist and requires a higher degree of client suitability than longer-term approaches (Safran, Segal, Shaw, & Vallis, 1990).

General Features of Cognitive-Behavioral Treatment for IBS

The general goal of cognitive-behavioral treatment for IBS is to help the client develop a reconceptualization of his/her bowel symptoms. This reconceptualization should shift from a view of IBS as a medical problem that is all encompassing and uncontrollable to a belief that the IBS symptoms (at least partially) are subject to the client's control. The purpose of all of the cognitive-behavioral procedures and treatment strategies is to develop these reconceptualized beliefs about more adaptive ways of coping with IBS.

The cognitive-behavioral approach to intervention is designed to be optimistic, emphasizing the client's ability to alleviate much of his/her IBS and/or distress associated with IBS. Throughout the intervention, IBS is reconceptualized so that the client comes to view his/her situation as amenable to change by means of a psychologically based approach. The treatment teaches the client a range of coping skills to assist him/her in dealing with unhelpful thoughts and feelings as well as noxious sensations that may facilitate or exacerbate symptoms. The cognitive-behavioral treatment relies heavily on active client participation and emphasizes a collaborative, problem-solving approach between client and therapist. In this manner, problems, concerns, and misunderstandings—in short, anything that can undermine successful treatment—are openly addressed throughout the intervention.

Cognitive-behavioral techniques are employed to facilitate the client to recognize and alter the association between thoughts, feelings, behaviors, environmental stimuli, and IBS symptoms. From this perspective, therapeutic gain is enhanced when the clients are actively involved and accept responsibility for examining the aspects of their own behavior that can be changed (Newman, 1994). Improvement is thus a function of both therapist and client efforts.

Treatment Objectives

To summarize, the cognitive-behavioral treatment approach can be viewed as having three major objectives:

1. To help the client to reconceptualize his/her view of IBS from helplessness and hopelessness to resourcefulness and hopefulness.
2. To help clients identify relationships among thoughts, feelings, behaviors, the environment, and IBS symptoms.
3. To empower clients to develop and implement increasingly more effective ways of coping with IBS in order to improve quality of life.

Representative Behavioral Intervention Strategies

As a rule, cognitive-behavioral treatment focuses on cognitive variables as targets of therapeutic change. Cognitive change, however, can be mediated by interventions targeting the behavioral components of functioning. These behavioral interventions may serve the larger goal of cognitive change in several ways. As one example, behavioral change, in and of itself, may interrupt the vicious cognition–affect–behavior cycle described earlier, thereby effecting synchronous change at the affective and cognitive levels. In cases where IBS is maintained by avoidant patterns (e.g., social withdrawal), behavioral interventions (e.g., exposure tasks) may serve to desensitize and provide evidence against catastrophic expectations (e.g., "Other people will laugh at me").

Thus, unlike strictly behavioral approaches to the treatment of IBS, cognitive-behavioral treatment employs behavioral strategies with the ultimate goal of addressing IBS-related cognitions. In the following sections, we highlight representative behavioral strategies. It should be emphasized that the selection of particular interventions should be guided by the therapist's conceptual formulation of the case. The willy-nilly application of "techniques" is a false caricature of cognitive-behavioral treatment and reflects a misunderstanding of its conceptual foundations.

Activity Scheduling

As noted earlier, behavioral activation can represent an important therapeutic goal, particularly in early phases of treatment. Clinicians can improve the likelihood of effective behavioral activation by working with clients to establish an activity schedule (see Lewinsohn & Graf, 1973). The first step in this process usually involves obtaining a baseline measure of clients' activities and corresponding moods. In the next phase, clients enumerate the tasks, responsibilities, and especially the pleasant activities they want to integrate into their schedules. Following this, a daily schedule can be worked out in which clients designate specific time slots for engaging in selected activities. These activities should include both pleasure- and mastery-related events. At this point, it can be helpful to have clients predict the amount of pleasure and/or mastery they expect to derive from each of the scheduled activities. In addition, obstacles to the successful completion of these activities should be anticipated and addressed, making contingency plans when possible. Finally, clients should be instructed to monitor their behavior, noting the actual degree of pleasure and/or mastery they derived from the scheduled activities. These actual pleasure and mastery ratings can be compared to clients' earlier ratings in order to obtain an index of the accuracy of their predictions.

Graded Task Assignments

In selecting and scheduling pleasant events and mastery tasks, it is important for therapists to attempt to maximize the likelihood of successful completion. As noted earlier, anticipating and dealing proactively with potential obstacles is one means of doing so. Another approach involves grading tasks such that clients start with the easiest tasks and then move on to greater challenges. Tasks may be simplified if they are broken down into smaller units. For example, whereas taking a long car trip with colleagues may represent an overwhelming prospect for a client with IBS, smaller components of the task, such as going for a short walk with a friend, may be more manageable.

Self-Reinforcement

Rewarding oneself for successfully accomplishing certain goals can represent an effective means of increasing levels of behavioral activation and of maintaining these gains. Therapists can encourage self-reinforcement by (1) providing a compelling rationale; (2) encouraging clients to establish specific, attainable goals with clearly defined performance criteria; (3) identifying activities that clients construe as reinforcing; (4) instructing clients to engage in reinforcing activities immediately after meeting their goals; and (5) monitoring clients' progress.

Representative Cognitive Intervention Strategies

The following are some representative strategies for addressing IBS-related thinking patterns. First, we focus on techniques for addressing automatic thoughts and unhelpful cognitions. Next, we consider strategies for dealing with the core beliefs, attitudes, and assumptions hypothesized to play a foundational role in the amplification of bowel symptoms.

Strategies Targeting Automatic Thoughts and Unhelpful Cognitions

DESIGNING EXPERIMENTS

In line with cognitive-behavioral treatment's emphasis on empiricism as a method, therapists typically encourage clients to regard their automatic thoughts as scientific hypotheses that then can be subjected to empirical (rather than strictly logical) examination. Automatic thoughts reported in the form of statements (e.g., "Having intestinal problems is a sign of weakness.") can usually be tested quite readily and, as such, make ideal hypotheses. However, automatic thoughts frequently are expressed in the form of questions (e.g., "Would I have these symptoms if I were stronger?"). In most cases, such queries can be translated into propositions via appropriate probes (e.g., "Do you have any thoughts about what having these problems means to you?", "What runs through your mind as you consider that question?", etc.).

Designing effective experiments can require a good deal of creativity and ingenuity on the part of both therapist and client. One means of generating ideas for experiments involves considering, a priori, the kind of evidence that could either support or disconfirm the hypothesis in question. To test the thought, "Having intestinal problems is a sign of weakness," for example, therapists and clients might first consider how the client defines the categories "weak" and "strong" in people, including the implications of being a "weak" or "strong" person. Next, an experiment could be designed in which clients might poll a random sample of acquaintances about the difference between a "weak" and

"strong" person. A series of such experiments could help undermine the subjective plausibility of clients' negative automatic
thoughts and might provide evidence for more helpful alternatives (e.g., "Many of the people I know seem to think about those
two terms in different ways than I do.").

OPERATIONALIZING NEGATIVE CONSTRUCTS

Automatic thoughts in IBS often have an absolutistic, black-and-
white quality. Examples of such thoughts are "I am a failure if I
embarrass myself in public" and "People will think I am a weak
person." The constructs (e.g., failure, weak person) that feature
so prominently in these negative automatic thoughts allow little
sense of gradation and, as such, can generate intensely negative
affect. One means of introducing some sense of gradation involves working with clients to operationalize these negative constructs. As a first step, clients are asked to provide specific, definitional criteria for the construct in question (e.g., "A failure is
someone who cannot exert self-control in any situation"). Next,
therapists can work with clients to construct a Likert-type scale
(e.g., a "failure" scale) to use to rate the extent to which they, and
other people they know, meet the definitional criteria identified
earlier. Most typically, these ratings will fall into the intermediate
range (i.e., denoting that the client has some vulnerabilities, but
that they are situational). As a result, clients may find that they
do not meet their own criteria for the negative label. More reasonable self-referential thoughts can then be considered (e.g., "I
am not a failure, but a human being who, like everyone else, can
cope in some situations but has difficulties in others."). Clients
can practice this approach whenever they notice themselves
thinking in terms of these absolute negative constructs.

CONSEQUENTIAL ANALYSIS

Clients with IBS often exhibit dramatic downward mood shifts in
response to what appear to be relatively benign automatic
thoughts. Consequential analysis (also known as the inverted ar-
row technique) can be a useful means of eliciting the underlying

fears, thoughts, or assumptions that may be generating an intense affective response. When employing this technique, therapists guide clients through a series of "What if . . . ?" questions. To illustrate, a client with IBS might report the automatic thought, "I feel anxious." When asked about the potential consequences of feeling anxious ("So, what if you are anxious?"), the client might respond, "It means something's wrong with me." The consequences of this, in turn, might be, "I'm abnormal," "No one will want to be with me," "I'll be rejected," or ultimately, "I will always be alone." Working with clients to make these links explicit can help them get a better understanding of their affective discomfort and reinforce the relationship between thoughts and feelings. Furthermore, the underlying assumptions (e.g., "When people feel anxious, it means there is something wrong with them.") can themselves be translated into hypotheses that may then be subjected to empirical test.

REATTRIBUTION

As noted earlier, automatic thinking in IBS is often associated with unhelpful patterns of attribution. Williams (1992) mentions a procedure in which clients imagine a hypothetical negative event (e.g., your stomach gurgles during a business meeting) and describe their naturally occurring attributions (e.g., "Everyone has heard my stomach," "They are all watching me now, judging me as having a problem with my digestion," etc.). Reasonable alternative explanations can then be generated and evaluated with respect to plausibility (e.g., "People do not notice these things if they are busy working on other matters," "It has happened to others in the room as well."). This technique can be rehearsed using actual events with an ultimate goal of enabling clients to (1) identify and monitor their unhelpful attributional patterns, and (2) develop proficiency in generating helpful alternative accounts of troubling events.

Strategies Targeting Unhelpful Core Beliefs

Changes at the level of automatic thoughts and unhelpful cognitions can effect rapid and marked symptomatic improvement. However, remission is likely to be short-lived when therapy has failed to address the enduring beliefs, rules, and attitudes that underlie IBS. Thus, whereas early stages of cognitive-behavioral treatment focus primarily on behavioral activation and change at the level of automatic thoughts, later sessions typically are devoted to addressing these more enduring cognitive elements.

HISTORICAL EXPLORATION

Despite their predominantly here-and-now orientation, some cognitive-behavioral theorists have suggested that unhelpful core beliefs or rules may have their origins in early experience. Examining the developmental roots of these beliefs can serve to weaken their present hold on the client in several ways. Most importantly, historical explorations can promote decentering—a process through which individuals, as it were, step outside of their immediate experience to view themselves engaged in constructing reality. Decentering "fosters a recognition that the reality of the moment is not absolute, immutable, or unalterable, but rather something that is being constructed" (Safran & Segal, 1990, p. 117). By examining how they have come to believe what they do, clients may come to regard their beliefs in a more tentative, less axiomatic fashion.

Furthermore, unhelpful beliefs often derive from interpretations of painful early experiences. In reviewing those circumstances, clients may recognize the reason behind these interpretations and work to revisit them. To illustrate, an individual with the core belief, "If someone criticizes me, then it means that I am a bad person," reported memories of being harshly criticized and punished by her father. In exploring these circumstances, she recalled attributing the father's attacks to her own badness, since, as a child, she could conceive of no other explanations for his hostile behavior. Her core belief was weakened when, as an adult, she was able to make alternative attributions for her father's behavior (e.g., he was under financial and personal pressure, had difficulty showing affection, was an ineffective father, etc.).

COST–BENEFIT ANALYSIS

As core beliefs are identified and challenged, therapists may be surprised to discover that clients can be reluctant to give them up. Often, this is due to the fact that the beliefs or rules have served a self-protective function or provided some important benefits. To illustrate, perfectionistic core beliefs (e.g., "If you can't do something perfectly, then don't bother doing it at all") can motivate impressive achievements. Clients are often loath to tamper with such beliefs, fearing that doing so may result in mediocrity or failure. In such cases, the costs and the benefits of maintaining such a belief system can be enumerated and compared. Similar cost–benefit analyses should be conducted on alternative but more helpful beliefs (e.g., "It's good to do as well as possible, but I can still enjoy something even if it's not perfect.").

RULE-BREAKING EXPERIMENTS

Core beliefs are commonly articulated in the form of general rules (e.g., "To be average is to be a contemptible nobody," "People will reject you if you make a mistake," etc.). Unfortunately, individuals with IBS rarely, if ever, expose themselves to the possibility of disconfirming evidence. Another approach to addressing these beliefs, therefore, is to design experiments in which clients deliberately seek out opportunities to break these fundamental rules and note the outcomes. Burns (1981) has provided a good example of an experiment designed to test the perfectionistic notion that being average leads to mediocrity and rejection. Here, clients are asked to make an effort to be as average as possible for a given period of time (e.g., 1 week). They typically discover, contrary to expectation, that this experience has no untoward effects; many even find it enjoyable. The ultimate goal, of course, is to weaken core beliefs by providing disconfirming evidence.

HELPFUL RESPONSES

The goal of cognitive restructuring is to teach participants to dispute their negative automatic thoughts with more empowering,

less anxiety-producing responses. Unlike Ellis and others, we pre-
fer the term "helpful responses" to "rational responses." Helpful
responses are not exercises in "looking at the bright side" or
thinking only good thoughts. Rather, helpful responses serve as
reminders that it is possible to cope with challenging life events
successfully.

Helpful responses do not deny the reality reflected in the
negative automatic thought (the "grain of truth"), but seek to
recontextualize and decatastrophize such thoughts and perceptions.

THE CALM METHOD

The CALM method of constructing helpful responses (Emmott,
1994) can help with the process of cognitive restructuring. It is
usually fairly difficult for participants to construct helpful responses when they first begin the process, perhaps because they
tend to have a low degree of belief in their own self-efficacy.
CALM is a mnemonic in which C stands for Consequences, A is
for Alternatives, L is for Logical Evidence, and M is for Meaning.

Consequences. The notion of consequences refers to the
evaluation of whether a particular thought or belief is helpful
and makes one feel better (more able to cope, less anxious and
depressed) or worse (more anxious, less able to cope). The
emphasis here is that individuals can have some power over what
they choose to believe. For example, if someone is cut off on the
highway, the thought, "I'd like to kill that stupid jerk—he's ruined
my good mood" has very different consequences than the
thought, "There goes another idiot in a hurry—I'm glad that I
have enough maturity to not get my kicks out of silly games in
cars."

Paying attention to the consequences of mood, symptoms,
and a sense of being in control can help to determine which particular automatic patterns of thought make things worse or make
things better.

The notion of assessing consequences of thinking patterns implies that making choices about how one interprets reality is an alternative to blind, unquestioning acceptance of negative thoughts as if they are gospel.

Alternatives. In order to construct helpful responses, it is useful to consider different possible interpretations of events. For example, if you were not included in a lunch with friends, some automatic thoughts are the following:

"They were deliberately excluding me."
"I did something to antagonize one of them."
"They have decided I'm not really any fun."

Alternatively, you might consider:

"This get-together was just for the people on the bowling
    league."
"They meant to invite me but forgot to call me."
"They know I'm vegetarian and were going to a steakhouse."
"Just because I don't do everything with that group doesn't
    mean they don't like me."

Obviously, some of these alternatives have negative consequences for self-esteem, while others serve to diminish the personal sting of being ignored. At the very least, considering that there may be alternative explanations leaves the door open to looking for additional information before the subject is closed.

One of the illustrations of the usefulness of looking for alternatives is to ask clients to recollect personal episodes of conflict in which they have felt that the other person failed to consider or appreciate their point of view. Such experiences are so common, and the failure of others to take the elementary steps to learn their point of view is so annoying, that clients may come to acknowledge the frequency with which they themselves wrongly assume they understand other people's motivations.

Logical Evidence. Logical evidence refers to looking for data or information so as to explore alternative explanations for ambiguous events. It is important that tangible evidence validate the assumptions on which behavior is based, because clients' willingness to engage in spontaneous or new behaviors is a function of the evidence that they marshal as to whether such efforts will be rewarding or successful. One of the traps in assembling evidence about the likelihood of success or failure in some endeavor is the overreliance on negative episodes in the past. This selective attention to distressing or unsuccessful attempts can be demoralizing and impede the willingness to engage in new behavior that is seen as "risky."

There are many methods of collecting evidence. The use of behavioral experiments based on progressive anxiety hierarchies can provide not only here-and-now counterexamples to past failures, but also vivid visual images of the individual succeeding in challenging, anxiety-producing situations. These images can be useful in constructing mental visualizations of successful responses to situations higher in the hierarchy.

Meaning. The final strategy for constructing helpful responses is to determine the personal meaning of an individual's specific automatic thoughts. It is not always clear why certain thoughts are more upsetting than others; people have unique areas of vulnerability which color their reactions to situations. For example, some persons may see the involuntary display of IBS symptoms such as stomach noises as exposing them to ridicule or the perception of others that they are not "genteel," while others may be concerned that they will be perceived as not sufficiently in control and therefore incompetent. For the former individuals, social ostracism may be feared, while the latter may be concerned that their authority will be questioned. Although all the individuals may experience similar levels of distress, the source of that distress, and the nature of the intervention required to address it, can vary considerably.

Often, the underlying meaning of events is not immediately apparent, or it may be highly idiosyncratic. It is useful to probe for additional automatic thoughts or underlying belief systems that might illuminate the emotional impact of events. Questions such as "What would it mean if ____ were to happen?" or "What is the source of the threat here?" are useful in ascertaining meaning.

HOT THOUGHTS

Greenberger and Padesky (1995) discuss the concept of "hot" automatic thoughts, which are those thoughts strongly connected to emotions. Often, these hot thoughts are connected to underlying critical self-statements. The authors' technique has clients rate each of their automatic thoughts in terms of the intensity of the negative mood associated with that particular thought, using a 1–100% scale. For example, if an individual felt an urgent need to pull off the highway to look for a bathroom while driving to a sales appointment with a colleague, she might be able to identify a number of thoughts and their associated moods: "This may make us late for our appointment" (anxious, 60%); "The bathroom we find may be dirty" (apprehension, 30%); and "My colleague is going to think that there's something wrong with me, that I'm weird" (anxious, 80%). The thoughts can then be ranked in terms of the intensity of emotion, from "cool" to "hot." In this example, the fear of being seen as weak or inadequate by a colleague, because of the threat to self-esteem, produces more anxiety (is "hotter") than concern about lateness or an unclean facility.

Greenberger and Padesky suggest selecting the automatic thought that is associated with the highest negative mood levels and searching for evidence that (1) supports that thought, and (2) does not support that thought. They note that in order to make this process credible to the client, it is important to look for evidence that supports both sides of the issue. Clinical experience suggests that personal evidence that is accessible to the client tends to be the most persuasive. The evidence that runs counter to the automatic thought does not necessarily have to be overwhelmingly persuasive; often, the mere existence of evidence not supporting the hot thought is enough to open the door to the possibility of alternative interpretations of events. For individuals who tend to use black-and-white thinking patterns, just the possibility of the existence of less rigid thinking patterns can be very helpful.

Group versus Individual Format

The treatment described in this book has been tested using a group format. But it may also be adapted for use with individuals. There are advantages and disadvantages to each format.

Group Format

In addition to being more cost-effective, there are further advantages in using a group format with a cognitive-behavioral treatment approach. For example, the efficacy of cognitive-behavioral group therapy for depression has been well documented (Gioe, 1975; Shaw, 1979; Taylor & Marshall, 1977; Rush & Watkins, 1981; Covi & Primakoff, 1988). As previously noted, a substantial number of clients with IBS also meet criteria for depression. Cognitive-behavioral therapy in a group format has been compared to an individual format in two controlled studies (Rush & Watkins, 1981). These studies demonstrated that the group format is as effective as the individual format in reducing depression (Rush & Watkins, 1981) and anxiety. The multiperson interactive context that the group provides is a rich source for corrective feedback (Rose, Tolman, & Tallant, 1985).

Individual Format

There are several advantages in using an individual format. Since most clients with functional bowel disorders have not been in psychological therapy, they may not be inclined to share their feelings in a group; individual clients can start immediately, without waiting for a group to begin, and missing sessions is less of an issue, since it is easy to reschedule individual appointments. Since the dynamics of groups are dependent on the mix of people within the group, individual contact can be better tailored to the individual needs of the client. Since previous research reveals that a substantial percentage of clients with IBS seen in gastroenterology clinics may also meet criteria for depression and/or an anxiety disorder, it is important to establish with the client which cognitive-behavioral models will be most helpful in conceptualizing the interplay between anxiety and/or depressive disorders and IBS. Moreover, a further challenge that the therapist may face is that some clients with IBS also present with a variety of nongastrointestinal symptoms and/or syndromes including coughs, fatigue, headaches, tenderness, stiffness, gynecological and urinary symptoms, backache, and hay fever (Sandler, Drossman, Nathan, & McKee, 1984; Whorwell et al., 1986; Colgan et al., 1988). Other investigators have observed that several functional somatic disorders not only may share many clinical features but also may overlap with one another. Examples of possible comorbidity with IBS include chronic fatigue syndrome, fibromyalgia, temporomandibular disorder, headaches, premenstrual syndrome, and chronic pelvic pain. Since many of these disorders also include pain as a salient feature, cognitive-behavioral pain management techniques such as imagery, attention, and relaxation are worth exploring with individual clients.

In essence, since each client with IBS may also have various combinations of these disorders and symptoms, the advantage of the individual format is that the therapist can develop a formulation of the presenting problems specifically tailored to each client.

3

Considerations of Stigma and Gender Role in Treating IBS

Most of the published treatments for IBS have been taken from theoretical approaches developed for work with individuals who presented to mental health professionals with largely depression or anxiety-related problems. Little theoretical or empirical work has identified and integrated into treatment specific psychosocial issues of individuals with IBS. Consequently, to date, there are few psychological approaches tailored to the needs of this population. Our group was the first to adapt cognitive-behavioral principles to clients with IBS using a specific cognitive-behavioral model (Toner, 1994). Although preliminary data appear promising, further refinement of cognitive-behavioral techniques tailored specifically to clients with IBS are needed.

Specifically, there are two areas that need to be further developed and incorporated into treatment. The first area is the impact of social stigma on clients with the disorder. There is a great deal of cognitive and emotional distress associated with having a debilitating chronic illness in this society. Insufficient knowledge and lack of empathy contribute to substantial stigma. The second area is gender as a variable in treating clients with IBS, the majority of whom are women (Toner, 1994). We believe that the impact of gender role is an important area needing treatment attention.

Stigma Associated with Functional Somatic Syndromes

Nearly every medical specialty has identified a functional somatic syndrome. These syndromes are usually defined by physical symptoms that are unexplained by organic disease. The term "functional" implies a disturbance of physiological function rather than anatomical structure (Kirmayer & Robbins, 1991). "Functional" is often contrasted with "organic" and conceptualized as psychogenic and less "real" (Fabrega, 1991). As a result of the stigma associated with the term "functional," various labels have been used to describe functional somatic syndrome. Such labels have included somatic disorders, health anxiety, physical symptoms not explained by organic disease, unexplained medical symptoms, and psychophysiological disorders. IBS is one of the most common functional somatic syndromes to attract increased research and clinical attention during the last decade.

In Western societies in general, and in medicine in particular, there is a moral dimension to a functional somatic disorder. Underlying the dualistic metaphysics of Western medicine, illness is either attributed to impersonal causes and viewed as an accident that befalls the patient as victim, or it is viewed as having a psychological cause that is mediated by and potentially under the person's voluntary control (Kirmayer, 1990). The morally perjorative connotations of a functional somatic disorder often leave patients believing that their problems are treated as "not real" and due to a psychological or moral defect or weakness (Kirmayer & Robbins 1991). Women are especially attentive to the possibility that their symptoms are not being taken seriously, since research has found that disorders disproportionately prevalent in women are often trivialized or described as psychological in origin (Lips, 1997). Unfortunately, as seen in the previous statement, "trivialized" and "psychological" are often equated in our society. Accordingly, it is important to highlight that when persons with IBS are referred to a health professional, they may come into the office with the belief that the caregiver does not think their symptoms are "real" or serious, but that they are "all in their heads." The therapeutic alliance is enhanced by validating the reality of the symptoms and also challenging society's view of the artificial dualism of functional/organic components of illness. Another area that needs to be considered is the influence of gender on IBS. For example, despite the repeated documentation of gender differences in clients with IBS (a ratio of three women to every man), there has been little attention devoted to gender issues in the conceptualization and treatment of IBS (Toner, 1994). The following section highlights the importance of including gender as a variable in therapy with clients with IBS.

Gender as a Variable in Therapy

Gender-Role Socialization and Role Conflict

There are a number of reports on treating gender as an important variable in cognitive-behavioral therapies (Davis & Padesky, 1989; Worell & Remer, 1992), but there is no discussion of gender in the cognitive-behavioral treatment of IBS. As summarized by Davis and Padesky (1989), it is particularly crucial to incorporate issues of gender into cognitive-behavioral treatment, since research suggests that gender plays a role in influencing individuals' reactions to various situations, as well as how they perceive themselves and are perceived by others (Deaux, 1984).

Moreover, one's gender can influence the development and organization of other schemas (Markus, Crane, Bernstein, & Siladi, 1982). For instance, several writers have suggested that in some fundamental ways, women experience a different social reality than men (Blechman, 1984; Resick, 1985; Shaef, 1985). Accordingly, certain content areas require added focus in therapy because of the relevance to women's social context. We have identified several salient content areas in the lives of women diagnosed with IBS. These fall under the general themes of gender-role conflict; physical functioning; relationship issues concerning nurturance, assertion and pleasing others; and physical, sexual, and emotional abuse. We first look at some features of gender-role socialization and conflict.

The importance of gender-role socialization in the expression of psychological disorders has received little attention within mainstream psychiatry and clinical psychology (Franks & Rothblum, 1983; Kelly, O'Brien, & Hosford, 1981; Lott, 1991). While the onset and maintenance of many disorders can be traced to complex interaction among several factors that could be experienced by either sex, in modern culture, women may be more vulnerable to these disorders since they are more likely to be confronted with conflicting messages regarding their gender role (Bepko & Krestan, 1990; Davis & Padesky, 1989; Worell & Remer, 1992).

Gender roles, which are socially prescribed attitudes, characteristics, and behaviors traditionally assigned to each sex, are acquired during development through differential treatment of boys and girls by parents, teachers, and societal institutions. Gender roles are based on socially shared beliefs that individuals should have certain qualities based on their biological sex. For example, the role of masculinity means one is instrumental and competency-oriented, and includes such traits as independence, rationality, competitiveness, and objectivity. The role of femininity means that one is expressive and relationship oriented, and it includes such traits as dependence, intuition, submissiveness, and emotionality (Lips, 1997).

Historically, the acquisition of sex-typed behaviors and characteristics, masculine and feminine identities, has been considered a prerequisite for mental health (Broverman, Broverman, Clarkson, Rosenkrantz, & Vogel, 1970). However, in our society, the female gender role is not compatible with what mental health professionals consider to be a healthy, mature adult (Broverman et al., 1970; Chesler, 1972; Pyke, 1985). In fact, highly sex-typed behaviors in women have been traditionally associated with anxiety, low self-esteem, and poorer emotional adjustment (Cosentino & Heilburn, 1964; Gall, 1969; Sears, 1970; Kleinplatz, Mccarrey, & Kateb, 1992). Thus, women in modern culture appear to be in a "double-bind" situation whereby in order to be seen as psychologically adjusted, they are encouraged to fulfill a gender role that is counterproductive to psychological well-being.

Other research suggests that women indeed experience confusion regarding the feminine gender role. A study by Gilbert, Deutsch, and Strahan (1978) suggests that while there is relatively little confusion regarding the ideal man for both sexes, there is confusion regarding the ideal woman. The confusion focuses on the extent to which male characteristics should ideally characterize a woman. For female participants, the ideal woman must somehow incorporate feminine and masculine characteristics simultaneously. Since these sex-typed characteristics are often contradictory and mutually exclusive (Feather & Simon, 1975), this finding is suggestive of gender-role conflict in women.

Attempting to incorporate both masculine and feminine behavior into one's gender role may promote gender-role conflict, because the two types of behavior may be incompatible (Steiner-Adair, 1986; Barnett; 1986). Indeed, sex-typed characteristics are often contradictory and mutually exclusive (Feather & Simon, 1975). For example, independence and assertiveness are two of the most prominent features of the male gender concept, whereas dependence and submissiveness are common themes in the female gender concept (Lips, 1997).

Perhaps the reason that women may feel pressure to incorporate both masculine and feminine traits into their gender role is that there is a contradiction between the behavior that is reinforced in women and that which is valued by society. Because gender roles are cultural standards prescribed for each sex, people are reinforced for adhering to their gender role and viewed as deviant if they do not (Lips, 1997). Thus, women are rewarded for developing characteristics that are congruent with their gender role, such as compliance, submissiveness, passivity, and weakness (Miller, 1987). However, as mentioned previously, masculine and not feminine sex-typed behavior has long been considered conducive to mental health and adjustment (Broverman et al., 1970) and therefore more highly valued by society. Thus, in contrast to men who are reinforced for behavior that is valued by society, and consistent with their gender role, women receive confusing information from society about the type of behavior that is expected from them.

This may translate into pressure for women to incorporate

both the highly regarded attributes of the masculine gender role and the prescribed feminine-typed behavior into their gender-role concept. However, it is difficult for women simply to adopt masculine traits, because females are rewarded for conforming to the feminine role (Long, 1991). In fact, it has been suggested that the expectation that women possess not only a number of feminine traits, but also masculine traits, can be stressful for women (Timko, Striegel-Moore, Silberstein, & Rodin, 1987). Consequently, women may experience a form of pervasive pressure to which men are seldom exposed, and that may predispose them to certain patterns of mental illness (Fodor, 1974; Franks & Rothblum, 1983).

In a world that is changing and becoming more demanding of women to perform not only relationally as wives and mothers, but also professionally as wage earners, this conflict is intensifying. Since masculine attributes are more highly valued, women may want to incorporate them, but in doing so, they run the risk of experiencing greater gender-role conflict. Feminine attributes are less valued, so men are less likely to aspire to them. Thus, gender-role conflict may be seen as a potentially more relevant issue for women than for men in our present society.

Admitting weakness, especially psychological vulnerability, is not socially desirable in our Western culture. Clients with IBS score higher on measures of social desirability than psychiatric and non-clinical groups (Toner, Garfinkel, Jeejeebhoy, Scher, et al., 1990). This could result in a gender-role socialization conflict among women seeking consultation for IBS symptoms. IBS has recently received the dubious label of "career woman's disease" in the popular press (Sandmaier, 1991). Female clients suffering from functional gastrointestinal disorders have been found to be more ambitious in terms of work and career goals than a nonclinical community sample of women (Craig & Brown, 1984). Abbey and Garfinkel (1991) have suggested that women who present with chronic fatigue syndrome often feel conflicted about the difficulty in balancing career, family, and personal wishes. We would suggest that vulnerability to certain expressions of psychological distress through physical symptoms may be related to difficulties in dealing with contradictions between interpersonal and achievement-oriented concerns in individuals with perfectionistic ideals. It is possible that while an overly pronounced focus on either of these areas of life events may lead to emotional distress (Beck, 1976), focusing on, and attempting to reconcile, their inherent contradictions may lead to a conflict that may be psychologically unhealthy as well. We are in the process of developing a gender-role socialization scale that taps into the messages women experience that may act as risk factors in the expression of certain patterns of psychosocial distress and bodily symptoms (Toner et al., 1999).

In a recent study (Ali, Richardson, & Toner, 1998), we investigated the association between the feminine gender role and illness behavior in IBS. We found the stereotypically feminine traits of submissiveness and passivity in women to be strongly related to disease conviction. Disease conviction is a mode of illness behavior that is characterized by affirmation that a physical disease exists, symptom preoccupation, and rejection of a physician's reassurance. It thus appears that patients who are more likely to adhere to attributes of the traditional feminine gender role are also more likely to focus on and express to their physician the physiological aspects of their experience of a functional bowel disorder. These findings are consistent with previous research that suggests somatizing patients often invest many of their personal resources in nurturing others rather than attending to their own needs (Barsky et al., 1988; Moldofsky & Lue, 1993). However, further research is required in order for us to more clearly understand the association between adopting the feminine gender role and experiencing symptoms of functional bowel disorders.

Physical Functioning

Davis and Padesky (1989) have identified common thoughts in women clients concerning body functioning. These frequently involve concerns over losing control, doing something socially unacceptable, appearing less than perfect, having something physically wrong with one's body, and not being able to control bodily functions through thoughts or behavior. A common clinical presentation is a hypervigilance or hyperawareness of any notable body sensation, with corresponding hyperconcern over the potential meaning of that sensation (Davis & Padesky, 1989). Men as well as women may be subject to developing these thoughts and attitudes. However, girls undergo a socialization process that is more likely to emphasize appearance, self-control, and restraint in physical activity (Davis & Padesky, 1989). Physical appearance and function have a great impact on a woman's sense of social worth. Davis and Padesky advise that an enhanced understanding of a woman's dysfunctional thoughts about her body functioning can be gained by recognizing that there is social and cultural reinforcement of the dysfunctional process. For example, while belching and passing gas are not usually socially desirable in public for either sex, girls and women are socialized into believing that they are especially not "ladylike" (e.g., "belching and farting" contests are less frequent among female than male adolescents). Moreover, bowel functioning is considered a taboo subject for "polite" conversation, and talking about associated symptoms is viewed as being in poor taste, embarrassing, and even shameful.

Davis and Padesky (1989) suggest that several underlying beliefs consistently reemerge across various areas of physically linked experiences among women. First, physical appearances are more important than physical functions. Physical functions are viewed as a source of embarrassment, devaluation, or loss of control. We have identified a number of these dysfunctional cognitions in our cognitive-behavioral groups with women with a diagnosis of IBS who have been referred to us from gastroenterologists (Toner et al., 1998). The most common IBS-related thoughts center around (1) public embarrassment and humiliation, and (2) perfectionistic or rigid views of bodily functions.

Self-Nurturance

As reviewed by Toner and Akman (1999), personality characteristics traditionally associated with femininity have significant implications for the expression and maintenance of IBS symptoms in women, as well as for their quality of life. Nurturance has been identified as a female trait, leading to the belief that women naturally gravitate toward taking care of others before taking care of themselves. This has led to the societal belief that it is wrong or unimportant for a woman to place priority on herself except in the interest of making herself more attractive to others (Davis & Padesky, 1989). Thus, women often spend their lives attending to the needs of their families, friends, and even coworkers, feeling guilty or selfish if they express a need of their own (Bepko & Krestan, 1990). This is important in the treatment of clients with IBS in two major ways. First, there should be some attempt to explore whether some of the symptoms women experience are related to stress, including the stress of taking care of their families while receiving little support for themselves. Health care professionals often assume that women are supposed to be taking care of others, and so rarely call this into question, more often preferring to view a woman's paying job as a source of stress. Women need to be encouraged to include themselves among those whom they are nurturing. Second, the clinical interpretation of women clients with IBS as needy and demanding is often a misinterpretation of the client's presentation. For many women, the expression of distress about their gastrointestinal symptoms and the demand for treatment may represent a very rare occurrence in their lives: They are acknowledging their own needs as well as a wish for support. Though they may communicate these needs in ways that physicians experience as demanding and difficult, this may provide an opportunity to reinforce these patients for taking good care of themselves. Thus, these patients may need to show more behaviors such as asking for help, taking time for themselves, and paying attention to not only their bodies, but also to their cognitions, emotions, and life stressors. In fact, Barsky et al. (1988) suggest that clients with "unexplained medical symptoms" (including IBS) are often quite surprised to realize how poorly they nurture themselves and often go out of their way to be helpful and supportive of other people's needs.

In our study of the relationship between the feminine gender role and illness behavior in IBS (Ali et al., 1998), it was evident that the clients who reported being more submissive to the demands of others were more likely to focus on the physiological symptoms of their condition. It is thus possible that individuals who nurture others rather than themselves may not be attuned to their own psychological or emotional needs. At the same time, however, individuals with severe IBS are forced by their gastrointestinal symptoms to be aware of their physical difficulties. Their symptoms may also be exacerbated the more they neglect nurturing themselves. Consequently, they may be hindered in seeing the connection between their own self-neglect, the resulting stress, and the impact on IBS symptoms. Thus, the psychological component of IBS may not be apparent to the individual with functional bowel symptoms, and the focus on the physical aspects of the disorder may become more prevalent.

Another component of self-neglect is self-blame, or taking responsibility for negative events. Women in our society are socialized to hold themselves responsible for things that go wrong in their lives and in the lives of people around them (Worell & Remer, 1992). Consequently, women report high levels of self-blame (Janoff-Bulman, 1979). In a recent study (Ali & Toner, 1996a), we examined the relationship between self-blame and IBS. We found that our sample of women with IBS reported significantly more self-blame than did our comparison group of women with inflammatory bowel disease. This study suggests that taking responsibility for negative events is more strongly associated with functional bowel disorders that organic bowel disorders.

Assertiveness, Need for Approval, and Pleasing Others

As previously discussed, gender-role socialization has encouraged girls and women to be nonassertive, putting others' needs before their own and not expressing anger, and being attuned to other people's feelings. One consequence of this differential gender-role socialization is that women more often than men have problems with anger and assertiveness. Common underlying schemas that have been identified by Davis and Padesky (1989) and Bepko and Krestan (1990) in their women clients are central themes with women diagnosed with IBS. These include: "I don't have a right to push my opinion on others," "It's better to please others and selfish to please myself," "Others always come first," and "It's not ladylike to raise your voice or show anger."

According to Major (1987), when individuals feel powerless or their needs are not being met, angry feelings are evoked. In the absence of "permission" to express these needs directly, women are likely to be more critical and self-blaming (Worell & Remer, 1992). Moreover, even when women behave in an appropriately assertive manner, it is often perceived by others as aggressive or inappropriate based on gender-role expectations. The relationship among the need to please others, expression of anger, assertiveness difficulties, and self-esteem needs to be explored and reframed in the context of gender-role socialization rather than being viewed as a personal deficit.

One gender-related schema that is associated with the expectation that women should focus on pleasing others is the self-silencing schema (Jack, 1991). According to the model of self-silencing, women adopt a self-silencing schema based on social expectations of what is required for a woman to create and maintain safe, intimate relationships. Such expectations can lead women to silence certain thoughts, feelings, and actions, which in turn can precipitate an overall self-negation through progressive devaluation of their own thoughts and beliefs.

Jack and Dill (1992) outline four basic components to self-silencing in women. The first is "externalized self-perception," which means judging the self by external standards. The second, "care as self-sacrifice," involves securing attachments by putting the needs of others before the self. The third component, "silencing the self," involves inhibiting one's self-expression and action to avoid conflict and possible loss of relationship. Finally, "the divided self" refers to the experience of presenting an outer self to live up to feminine role imperatives while the inner self becomes resentful of being silenced. These four components are grounded in the context of intimate relationships as well as the societal expectations of women.

High levels of self-silencing have been demonstrated in a number of different populations of women. These include women residing in battered women's shelters and mothers (of 4-month-old infants) who reported cocaine use during pregnancy (Jack & Dill, 1992). Self-silencing also has been found to correlate significantly with depressive symptomatology in depressed as well as control group women (Jack & Dill, 1992). In a recent study

(Ali & Toner, 1996b), we compared a sample of 25 women diagnosed with IBS to 25 women diagnosed with organic bowel disease. We found self-silencing to be significantly more prevalent in the women with IBS than in the women with the organic bowel disease. These findings suggest a specific association between functional bowel symptoms and the societal demands on women to put the needs of others before their own needs.

Physical, Sexual, and Emotional Abuse

A history of abuse in childhood or adulthood has been identified as a risk factor for women in the development of a number of psychiatric disorders, including depression, eating disorders, anxiety, somatoform disorders, borderline personality disorder, and dissociative disorders (Beitchman et al., 1992; Browne & Finkelhor, 1986; Greenwald, Leitenberg, Cado, & Tarran, 1990; Walker, Gelfand, Gelfand, Koss, & Katon, 1995). Studies examining the relationship between sexual or physical abuse and health status reveal that women who have experienced abuse are significantly more likely than nonabused women to present to physicians with complaints of pelvic pain, headaches, backaches, fatigue, and joint pain (Domino & Haber, 1987; Walker et al., 1988). Women with sexual or physical abuse histories have also been shown to have had significantly more lifetime surgeries, hospitalizations, and physician visits than their nonabused counterparts (Drossman et al., 1990). All of these findings point to the importance of investigating an association between functional bowel disorders and history of abuse.

A number of recent investigations have examined the relationship between a history of physical and sexual abuse and gastrointestinal illness (Drossman et al., 1990; Felitti, 1991; Longstreth & Wolde-Tsadik, 1993; Rimsza, Berg, & Locke, 1988). Along with genitourinary symptoms, gastrointestinal symptoms are the most common complaint of female children who have experienced sexual abuse (Rimsza et al., 1988). Also, among women seen in primary care settings, gastrointestinal complaints are the most common somatic symptoms reported by women with a history of physical or sexual abuse (Felitti, 1991; Lechner, Vogel, Garcia-Shelton, Leichter, & Steibel, 1993). Specifically, Felitti (1991) reports in a study of general practice clinics that 64% of women reporting a history of physical and/or sexual abuse complained of gastrointestinal symptoms compared to 39% of women reporting no abuse history. It should further be noted that women seen at referral centers by gastroenterologists report higher rates of physical and sexual abuse than do women seen in primary care settings (Drossman et al., 1990; Longstreth & Wolde-Tsadik, 1993).

Studies of relative prevalence rates in clients with organic bowel disease compared to clients with functional bowel disorders report high abuse rates in clients with IBS (Walker, Katon, Roy-Burne, Jemelka, & Russo, 1993; Drossman et al., 1990). Walker et al. (1993) found that 54% of clients with IBS reported a history of sexual abuse relative to a 5% prevalence rate in clients with inflammatory bowel disease. In a review, Laws (1993) reported that a history of sexual abuse occurs with high frequency in women with functional bowel disorder. Similarly, Drossman et al. (1990) found that clients diagnosed with functional bowel disorders were significantly more likely than were clients with organic bowel disorders to have had a history of forced intercourse and to have experienced frequent physical abuse. Leserman et al. (1996) found that female clients with functional gastrointestinal disorders were significantly more likely than control group female clients to have been victims of rape and to have experienced life-threatening physical abuse. An abuse history in clients with gastrointestinal disorders contributes to poorer health status. These clients have (1) more severe pain, (2) more physical and psychosocial disability, (3) greater psychosocial difficulties, (4) higher health care use rates, and (5) more surgical procedures, and this is independent of diagnosis (Talley, Fett, Zinsmeister, & Melton, 1994; Drossman, Li, Leserman, Toomey, & Hu, 1996; Longstreth & Wolde-Tsadik, 1993; Drossman et al., 1990). Sexual abuse may act as a nonspecific (but particularly severe) psychological stressor that increases physiological arousal and thereby triggers or exacerbates gastrointestinal symptoms (Whitehead, 1998).

Despite such evidence regarding the prevalence of physical and sexual abuse, few studies to date have examined the impact of emotional abuse in IBS (Talley, 1996). Emotional abuse can be defined as any form of verbal statements of threat, denigration, or accusation, and behavior that is dangerous, threatening, or negligent (Briere & Runtz, 1990). In one study (Ali & Toner, 1996b; Ali et al., in press), we assessed the presence of emotional abuse in adulthood (persons older than age 14) in two samples of women diagnosed with IBS and inflammatory bowel disease, respectively. Using a quantitative questionnaire, we found that emotional abuse was significantly more prevalent in the women with IBS than in the women with organic bowel disorders. Furthermore, in response to a qualitative, semistructured interview, a large number of the women with IBS reported that they perceived past physical, sexual, or emotional abuse to play an important role in the precipitation and/or exacerbation of their bowel symptoms.

There is thus convincing evidence that physical, sexual, and emotional abuse are very prevalent in women diagnosed with IBS. Like self-blame, self-silencing, and high need for approval, the experience of abuse can be understood from a perspective of gender-role socialization. These empirical findings and clinical observations have implications for both the assessment and treatment of women who present with IBS. It is important to address these content areas in our understanding of societal expectations of women and to integrate this information and awareness into our cognitive-behavioral therapies.

The Integration of Feminist Therapy Principles with Cognitive-Behavioral Treatment

The integration of gender as a relevant variable in cognitive-behavioral treatment requires some understanding of feminist principles in therapy. The hallmark principles in feminist therapy are that (1) the personal is political, (2) relationships are egalitarian, and (3) women are valued. As summarized by Worell and Remer (1992), these principles are compatible with cognitive-behavioral theory and could be readily incorporated into cognitive-behavioral therapy. In practice, two modifications identified by Worell and Remer (1992) would increase both the compatibility with principles of feminist therapy and the efficacy of cognitive-behavioral therapy for women with functional somatic syndrome: (1) incorporation of social role theory, and (2) relabeling or reframing of pathologizing concepts in order to emphasize the social context.

SOCIAL ROLE THEORY

Of primary importance is the incorporation of social role theory into cognitive-behavioral therapy in order to further highlight the socialized role expectations and power imbalances that permeate individuals' lives (Worell & Remer, 1992). This addition would allow cognitive-behavioral therapies to interpret current cognitions and behavior in terms of gender-role socialization and conceptualize situational behavior within a broader societal context (e.g., patriarchy, sexism, discrimination, power imbalance). The integration of social role theory would also foster the use of concepts that describe aspects of role behavior such as gender-role conflict. Finally, social role theory would serve to relabel or reframe certain cognitive-behavioral concepts such as deficit behavior in terms of over- or undersocialization. Accordingly, more emphasis could be placed on resocialization or reconstructing environments rather than remediation and deficit behavior (Worell & Remer, 1992).

RELABELING PATHOLOGIZING CONCEPTS

A second modification to cognitive-behavioral therapy that would be facilitated by the integration of social role theory is the relabeling of certain cognitive concepts such as distortion, irrationality, and erroneous or faulty thinking. These concepts infer that individual pathology or idiosyncratic cognitions are a primary cause of the person's problem, while placing minimal emphasis on the social context. It is important to test the hypothesis that the client's perceptions and cognitions do match the realities of his/her life situation. For example, research has revealed that depressed individuals distort the objective world less than nondepressed individuals (Hammen, 1988).

THE INTEGRATION OF THE SOCIAL CONTEXT
IN COGNITIVE-BEHAVIORAL THERAPY: A CASE EXAMPLE

The following vignette highlights the need to incorporate the larger social context into an understanding of the issues presented:

> A. B. is a single, 39-year-old lawyer in a prominent law firm. She has experienced IBS for the past 5 years and has consulted several gastroenterologists to find out what is causing her unpredictable bouts of diarrhea and intense abdominal pain. She is convinced that something has been missed and that the doctors are not taking her seriously and are treating her like a "hysterical woman." In spite of her symptoms, she has never taken a day off and is considered by her colleagues and friends as always being "in control" and "on top of things." She describes herself as a very considerate person who will always go out of her way to help colleagues or friends, but recently, she is thinking that others are taking advantage of her. However, she finds it difficult to express any anger she may feel over this. Also, she seldom has time for herself and confesses that she has not taken a vacation in over 2 years.
>
> She describes herself as an ambitious person, but she feels somewhat dissatisfied with her career since she has not become a partner in the firm. She has seen junior people advance over her and wonders if she is doing something wrong. The few times that she has assertively stated her needs and expectations to her supervisors she has been met with resistance. Sometimes she feels that her ideas are not being taken as seriously as those of her male colleagues. She feels somewhat isolated at work, since she is one of the few women lawyers and the only single woman lawyer. She worries that she may never find a satisfying relationship and fears that with respect to having children, she is running out of time. Recently, she has felt increasingly depressed, tense, and exhausted.

In order to understand the client's "problem," it is important to explore the realities in her life as well as the possible "distortions" in her thinking. Moreover, it is important to check out whether A. B. is behaving, thinking, and feeling in accordance with her understanding of society's expectations for her (Worell & Remer, 1992). Rather than convince her of possible errors in thinking (e.g., "I may never find a satisfying relationship," "I'm a failure as a woman if I don't have children," "I'm a failure at work because I'm not a partner," "If I have difficulty being assertive and expressing anger, there must be something wrong with me," "Something must be missing since I have so much abdominal pain"), the therapist could explore societal messages about the "good woman" (i.e., a good woman marries and has children, never gets angry, puts others' needs before hers, never looks flustered or needy), stereotypes about single women (i.e., "old maid"), fears about living without a partner (i.e., women are helpless and need to be taken care of), and stereotypes about pain and organic cause (i.e., if it is "really" painful, there must be an organic etiology).

It is important to encourage clients like A. B. to monitor both their automatic thoughts and their sex-role messages. In this process, we can aid clients in understanding that regardless of external realities, some thoughts and behaviors are not helpful and can contribute to dysphoric moods and somatic distress. Accordingly, the principles of techniques such as cognitive restructuring can be implemented without using pathologizing labels and client-blaming attributes (Worell & Remer, 1992). The integration of feminist principles into cognitive-behavioral therapy shifts the focus to identifying and changing the unhealthy external situation and to identifying and changing the internalized effects of the external social context. We encourage therapists to use this framework throughout the course of cognitive-behavioral therapy with clients with IBS. This focus is especially important when discussing themes that are related to coping with IBS including shame, anger, assertion, self-efficacy, social approval, perfectionism, and control (see Chapter 7).

II

CLINICAL APPLICATION

4

Assessment

We recommend that routine assessment of clients with IBS for this treatment include a medical evaluation and a psychological interview that screens for psychiatric diagnosis and assesses baseline physical symptoms and illness cognitions. These areas, together with related assessment issues and recommendations, are described in this chapter. Note, however, that our research protocol did not include a session on assessment since pre- and posttreatment measures were given separately by a research assistant in order to keep the therapist blind to psychosocial changes during the course of therapy.

Medical Assessment

Persons suspected of having IBS should be evaluated initially by a gastroenterologist to rule out any pathological conditions and establish medically appropriate regimens. Medical conditions that should be ruled out through a medical workup include inflammatory bowel disease, intestinal parasites, lactose intolerance, or other gastrointestinal diseases. The criteria for establishing a diagnosis of IBS have been previously discussed. This diagnosis is based on identifying positive symptoms consistent with the condition and including other conditions with similar clinical presentation.

As documented in a recent position paper for the American Gastroenterological Association,

> A physical examination and the following studies are recommended for routine evaluation: complete blood count; sedimentation rate; chemistries; stool for ova, parasites, and blood; and flexible sigmoidoscopy or colonoscopy or barium enema with sigmoidoscopy if older than 50 years. Other diagnostic studies should be minimal and will depend on the symptom subtype. For example, in patients with diarrhea-predominant symptoms, a small bowel radiograph to rule out Crohn's disease, or lactose/dextrose H_2 breath test. For patients with pain as the predominant symptom, a plain abdominal radiograph during an acute episode to exclude bowel obstruction and other abdominal pathology. (Drossman et al., 1997, p. 2118).

Psychological Assessment

Following medical evaluation, the psychological assessment interview with the therapist takes place. As Salkovskis (1992) has pointed out, a fundamental principle of the cognitive-behavioral approach is that a psychological formulation in positive terms, rather than by exclusion, is the basis of a usable assessment upon which a treatment plan can be based. The formulation of a testable and understandable explanation of symptoms serves both to relieve the client's anxiety and concerns about being seen as having "imaginary" complaints, and to devise tests of working hypotheses based on the formulation, which can be modified in response to progress or lack of it.

Medical History/Symptoms

The medical history should be reviewed with the client. The client can be asked to give the narrative history of the condition and describe relevant psychosocial events surrounding the symptoms. The relative chronicity of the illness will affect its impact; chronic conditions often are associated with greater psychosocial concomitants, either contributing to or resulting from the medical condition. The client's perceptions of the course of the illness and its impact on her/his quality of life, relationships, and functional abilities are central in the therapist's formulation of the meaning of the illness to the client. During this interview, the therapist can begin to assess the client's relative openness to the assumptions underlying a cognitive model of treatment by asking the client if symptoms can be triggered by fatigue, diet, work pressure, or other stressors.

By the time clients with IBS have been referred to a therapist, they may feel discounted and suspect that their problems are not being seen as real. During the client's initial description of symptoms, the therapist has the opportunity to establish a collaborative bond with the client by validating his/her account of pain and distress as not imaginary or "all in the head." It is useful for the therapist to explore the client's interpretation of the referral in the process of developing a shared model of the problem. A symptom diary, a pain diary, or standardized scales can be used as assessment methods. Non-IBS physical symptoms should also be elicited.

Symptom Diary

While the IBS symptoms reported by the client are being reviewed, the therapist may find it helpful to introduce the Functional Bowel Disorders Diary Form (Drossman, 1995a; see Appendix 1). The diary has the client describe daily bowel movements and pain. Although most clients can be categorized in terms of symptoms primarily of diarrhea, primarily of constipation, or mixed diarrhea and constipation, some clients indicate that their distress is attributable mostly to pain, bloating, or gas. Ideally, clients should complete the symptom diary during a pretreatment phase and continue to use the diary form through the treatment phase. This will provide information that is useful for assessing progress and quantifying improvement.

Pain Management

The nature, duration, and intensity of the client's pain may be assessed through his/her descriptive reports, by use of a simple visual analogue scale, as included in the daily diary card, or by means of standardized scales, such as the McGill Pain Questionnaire.

Non-IBS Symptoms

In addition to the assessment of IBS symptoms, the therapist should also note the presence of other physical problems. A lifelong history of multiple physical symptoms, high rates of disability, multiple diagnostic procedures, or poorly explained physical conditions may alert the therapist to possible somatic patterns of expression of illnesses.

Psychiatric Diagnoses

Since the literature appears to establish a higher incidence of psychiatric comorbidity among individuals with IBS seen in tertiary settings, the current and lifetime prevalence of psychiatric disorders should be assessed, paying particular attention to diagnoses of anxiety, depression, and somatoform disorders.

Three types of instruments are used to assess psychiatric disorders. The first are structured research interviews, such as the Diagnostic Interview Schedule or the Structured Clinical Interview for DSM-IV, which assess the extent of specific symptoms of psychiatric diagnoses according to predetermined criteria. These measures tend to be extensive and highly time-consuming. The second are measures of psychological state, such as generic self-report screening instruments such as the Symptom Checklist 90–Revised or the General Health Questionnaire. High scores on these instruments are commonly associated with specific psychiatric diagnoses, which can be further documented through interviews. Third are syndrome-specific screening instruments that may be self-scored or interviewer-directed questionnaires assessing symptoms of specific psychiatric syndromes. These would include measures of depression, such as the Beck Depression Inventory, or anxiety, such as the Spielberger State–Trait Anxiety Scale (Spielberger, 1985). A combination of these measures, in conjunction with the clinical interview, can provide useful documentation to the clinician in establishing a psychiatric diagnosis.

In using psychometric assessment techniques, care must be taken not to base diagnoses on measures for which physical symptoms, especially gastrointestinal symptoms, are scored as indicating somatization, anxiety, or depression. The identification of Axis I disorders is important in treatment planning, since it is likely that concurrent treatment of the psychiatric disorder will be necessary in addition to treatment of IBS.

Social Context and Gender Issues

Certainly the social context of individuals with IBS has an impact on their experience of their illness and its treatment. The cognitive-behavioral perspective recognizes the role of sociopolitical environments in conjunction with the individual's perceptions of environmental events in maintaining and reinforcing problematic behaviors. Feminist therapy has adopted a similar perspective in its analysis of issues such as family violence and eating disorders. A number of gender issues may be relevant in IBS. Women's socialization for fastidiousness and social approval may increase the stigma of IBS and make women more vulnerable to anxiety about their symptoms being noticed by others. Women with a history of sexual or physical abuse appear to be substantially more at risk for IBS, and women may be reluctant to disclose this information to physicians. Exploration of abuse issues ought to occur as the therapist assesses the family and relationship history.

Gender issues may also emerge in clients' descriptions of their family and work responsibilities. Women with IBS often endorse the expectation that they should provide practical and emotional support to their families and work colleagues, and put their own needs for support last on their list of priorities. In addition, many women juggle multiple responsibilities at home and at work. Aside from the fact that individuals with multiple roles and stressors may have fewer physical and psychological resources to draw upon when they are under physical or psychological stress, women may be reluctant to acknowledge that they are worthy or deserving of self-care. They also may have fewer financial or personal resources to aid them in alleviating demanding responsibilities, and more perceived obligations to others.

Assessing Social Supports and Stressors

Therapists and researchers agree that, like other issues we face in our daily living, having a functional bowel disorder is likely both to impact and be impacted by our relationships with family and friends. To the degree that social and familial relationships are considered central in a person's life, they should be considered relevant avenues of exploration in treatment. Given that we are proposing a psychosocial approach to treatment for bowel disorders, we would be remiss if we did not address the different ways practitioners can work with clients to explore how their bowel disorder, interpersonal relationships, and the degree to which they feel supported may be linked. Relevant interpersonal relationships are considered those that clients have with spouses, family members, friends, or other associates that clients identify as being an important part of their lives (Akman & Toner, 1999).

While there are approaches to couple and family therapy that focus on the cognitions and behaviors of family members (see Falloon,1991; Holtzworth-Munroe & Jacobson, 1991), this section is not intended to provide an overview of psychotherapy for couples and families. Our intent is to help therapists and clients alike begin to think in systemic terms so that the clients and their bowel disorders are seen not in isolation but as part of a broader experience that includes other people with whom the client is interacting. We offer some suggestions for orienting clients to consider their health and well-being within the broader context of their lives, and we discuss some possibilities for including family and/or friends in actual treatment sessions. A major focus of this discussion is on facilitating a support system for people who suffer from bowel problems.

Thinking about Family and Friends

From the assessment stages to the completion of treatment, therapists need to be thinking and probing from a contextual perspective. Asking questions about a client's relationships is appropriate in the initial stages of treatment for engagement purposes and for exploring possible links between relationship issues and the bowel disorder, and to signify to clients that information about their relationships and the larger context in which they live is important and interesting. Clients in general, and particularly clients with medical complaints, are often used to thinking about their concerns in terms that minimize or exclude those things outside of themselves. It is important to help clients begin to contextualize their issues so that they can begin to think differently about where their bowel disorder fits into their lives. The goal is not to promote a "cause and effect" relationship among the clients, the bowel disorder, and their environment, but rather to help client gain some new perspective on the link between their physical symptomology and the external environment. Clients are often surprised to discover that the onset of the disorder, or changes in the intensity of their symptoms, sometimes coincide with important life events, such as marriage, divorce, the birth of a child, the death of a parent, relationship difficulties, or other stressors such as geographical moves or job changes (Craig & Brown, 1984; Creed et al., 1988; Drossman, 1995b).

If the client is involved in a relationship, the therapist might begin to explore how the bowel disorder fits into the relationship. Questions about the partner's knowledge of and reaction to the client's symptoms can elicit important information about the degree to which the client is sharing the experience as well as the degree to which he/she feels supported. Questions exploring the content and frequency of communication regarding the bowel symptoms can also prove to be useful in determining the impact the bowel disorder has had on the relationship, as well as the impact the relationship may have had on the bowel disorder. When one partner has a medical disorder, it is not unusual for couples to experience some impact on various aspects of their relationships, including their sex life, the division of household labor and parenting responsibilities, and their social lives (Rolland,1994). People also often report that aspects of their relationship can have an effect on their symptom frequency and intensity. Once the therapist and client have an understanding of some of the stressors and supports that exist for the client, therapy sessions should include an examination of these stressors and new ways of coping with them, as well as exploring and maximizing the client's support system (Akman & Toner, 1999).

Examples of Questions

Does your partner know about the bowel disorder? If so, what was his/her reaction? Has your partner's reaction changed over time? How does he/she currently respond to your symptoms?

How has the bowel disorder affected your verbal and physical expression of intimacy? Specifically, how has it affected your sexual relationship? Who is most bothered by the effect on your sex life?

What is the nature of the division of household and parenting responsibilities in your relationship? How has it changed over the years? What impact do you think these responsibilities have had on your symptoms? What impact do you think your bowel disorder has had on your abilities or desire to maintain your responsibilities? How has your relationship with your children been affected by your bowel disorder? What would your partner say to these questions?

If there were no bowel disorder, how might your home life be different?

Do extended family members and friends know about your bowel disorder? If so, how do they respond to you? Does anyone else in your family or circle of friends have a bowel disorder?

How do your family/partner/friends help you feel hopeful/hopeless about your bowel disorder? How do you help them feel hopeful or hopeless about your bowel disorder?

When to Invite Family/Friends into Therapy

Clearly not all clients will want or need to bring their family members or friends into therapy. Therapists should consider including family members and/or friends in therapy when (1) the client expresses a desire to have someone else attend one or more sessions as a way of sharing in the experience, or (2) the client identifies a person(s) who already is or potentially may be a source of support, and the session could be used as a forum to express gratitude for the ongoing support and to examine ways of facilitating any potential support.

It is important that both the therapist and client have a clear understanding of the purpose of inviting someone else into the session, and that this purpose is relayed to the person who is being asked to participate. When people are invited to attend someone else's therapy session, they often respond by being suspicious about why they are being asked to attend and worry that they will somehow be held to blame for the problem, or they are unclear about how their presence will be of use. The therapist and client can work together to formulate a plan for inviting this person, keeping in mind the nature of the relationship and the client's own knowledge of how this person is likely to respond to such a request.

Assessing Beliefs about Needing Support

Many people who suffer from debilitating medical ailments, including bowel disorders, experience worry or guilt about being a burden to those around them. This sometimes results in clients' reluctance to ask for, or feel worthy of receiving, the care and support that they may legitimately need. In addition, because having a bowel problem is such a shameful experience for many people, it is often kept hidden from the rest of the world, resulting in a vicious cycle of isolation and shame. The more one is ashamed, the more one retreats into isolation, and the more one is isolated, the stronger are the feelings of shame.

An important focus of therapy, therefore, should be to help the client to examine his/her beliefs about needing and asking for support, then identify those people he/she considers to be supportive, and finally to learn how to ask for and receive the support that is available (Akman & Toner, 1999).

EXAMPLES OF QUESTIONS

> Who in your life gives you the most support in coping with your bowel problems? What does this person do that you find supportive? Can you think of someone who has the most potential for being supportive? What makes you think that this person could possibly be supportive? Does this person know you consider him/her supportive or potentially supportive? Who do you wish would be more supportive? What do you think stops this person from showing you more support? What do you think this person needs in order to become more supportive?
>
> How do you respond when someone says or does something supportive? How does it make you feel to be supported?
>
> How do you let others know that you need support?
>
> What do you need more or less of from the people in your life? What do you think they need more or less of from you?
>
> What do you think you do that encourages people to show support? What do you think you do that discourages them?

Some clients will be unable to identify a source of support. It is important to determine whether this is because they are predicting that no one would be willing to support them, or because they truly do not have a system of support in place. In the case of the former, it would be important to examine and test the client's beliefs about the significant people in his/her life, while in the latter case, the therapist would need to work with the client to broaden his/her support system and to find someone who could be even minimally supportive. Some examples of potential sources of support might be a colleague in whom the client could confide, or a neighbor with whom to have tea or call on to run errands in case the client is ill. With clients who are unable to identify any sources of support, an important goal of therapy is to reduce the sense of isolation that is being experienced by helping the client to reconsider his/her current relationships and/or expand his/her social network as much as possible.

The issue of asking for and receiving support can be both foreign and threatening to many people for a multitude of reasons. People who have come to view themselves as caring for others, rather than caring for self, often have never entertained the idea they are someone who legitimately needs and deserves support from others. They also have trouble conceiving of the notion that they can and should be supportive of themselves. To be truly self-supportive means to allow room for flexibility, for flaws, for nurturance, and for fun, and many people abandon these notions for fear of feeling like a failure, for fear of public embarrassment and loss of control. With people who seem to be lacking support from others and tolerance from themselves, it may be necessary to begin by addressing the contribution that self-understanding and self-care can make to their emotional and physical well-being.

Clearly, one of the prerequisites to asking for support is knowing when and in what way one needs support. For instance, if a person is feeling fatigued, he/she would first need to recognize the fatigue, determine what would help alleviate some of the it, and then know how to go about getting that relief. Many people would find even the first step of identifying their experience as difficult. When a person is preoccupied with caring about others, worrying about his/her public presentation, and maintaining a very high degree of responsibility, self-awareness is often sacrificed. It is not uncommon to hear clients with functional bowel disorders claim that they simply do not know what they need most, from themselves or others, because they are too busy focusing on keeping their world orderly. The notion of support for self, therefore, is one that is given last place in their list of priorities, if it makes the list at all. A useful avenue to travel with these clients may be one that explores their understanding of themselves, their capacity to be multifaceted, both privately and publicly, and the degree to which they allow themselves to be fully functioning persons who at times need support. The following questions are designed to introduce and validate these ideas to people who are reluctant to allow themselves to need and then ask for support.

> When do you feel truly free from the responsibilities of
>   your life?
> What are you like when you are really being yourself?
>   When was the last time you were really yourself?
> When was the last time you acted silly or playful? How did
>   it feel? How do people around you respond when you
>   act that way? How do you respond when you see others
>   acting silly or playful?
> What would be the most frightening aspect of letting go
>   of some of your responsibilities? What would be the
>   nicest aspect of it?
> What is your idea of a perfect day? When was the last
>   time you had a perfect day?

Assessing Cognitions and Coping Style

The presence of unhelpful cognitions and cognitive styles, as commonly seen in individuals with IBS, has been identified by a number of researchers. Such styles include perfectionism, high need for approval, and a tendency to focus on the catastrophic nature of difficulties. Such styles make it difficult for clients to normalize their symptoms and tend to increase arousal and anxiety levels.

Recently, Toner et al. (1998a) developed a valid and reliable scale for assessing IBS-related cognitions. The Cognitive Scale for Functional Bowel Disorders measures both indicators of impairment in various situations (meetings, restaurants, traveling) and cognitions that tend to increase the distress of the individual with IBS (perfectionism, perceptions of IBS as abnormal or shameful, high need for control). This 25-item scale has been validated on samples of clients with IBS in Canada and the United States, and has been found to be strongly correlated with both symptomatic distress and other measures of anxiety and distress. An important facet of the development of this scale was the development of themes that capture the common concerns of clients with IBS. These themes were derived from a number of sources, including the thought diaries of clients, literature reviews, and the clinical and research experience of health care professionals involved in IBS. The themes were developed in order to address comprehensively the domain of cognitions relevant to clients with IBS. Therefore, the 25 items in our final scale are each related to a particular theme: bowel performance anxiety, control, social approval, perfectionism, anger, pain, self-efficacy, shame, and self-nurturance. The following chapters discuss these themes in detail, as well as provide clinical examples of how each theme may be represented in the lives of clients with IBS. We introduce these themes briefly here.

One key theme relevant to clients with IBS is that of *bowel performance anxiety*. This theme manifests itself in the worry that the bowels will not function or perform properly, and much attention is paid to managing food and environment to mimimize the likelihood of bowel distress. The case of B. C., a 37-year-old office worker, addresses this concern. This woman spent weeks worrying about upcoming office dinners, wishing she could somehow be excused from them. In order to try to manage her anxiety, she would visit the restaurant in advance of the dinner, checking the location of the washrooms, and determining which table would be best for her in case a quick visit to the washroom was necessary. Days before the dinners, she would restrict her food intake to ensure that her stomach would not be acting up, and at the dinners, she would limit herself only to those foods she was absolutely sure would be "safe."

Control is a prominent theme. This refers to the idea that since they are unable to control their bowels, clients with IBS often try to control as much of their environment as possible so as to avoid unpleasant and/or awkward situations. The experience of C. D., a 33-year-old woman with IBS, provides a telling example. C. D.'s main symptom was vomiting, and her concern was that she would vomit unexpectedly in public. To control this, she would only dine out at restaurants where tables were spaced far apart, affording diners some privacy, and only with certain people with whom she felt comfortable. Her reluctance to go to restaurants with various friends caused some problems in her relationships, and her insistence on eating at only certain establishments would sometimes contribute to a perception of her as being "difficult."

Another important theme to emerge is that of *social approval*, which refers to the idea that clients with IBS are often concerned with how they appear in the eyes of others, not wanting to present themselves as foolish or incompetent. K. L. was a 30-year-old woman who held a demanding job in an accounting firm. Though she was presenting for treatment for IBS, she was reluctant to share with the therapist some of the difficulties she was experiencing. She admitted that she worried about what people would think of her, and, in fact, she had not shared with her coworkers anything about her bowel problems, lest they think she could not handle her job.

Linked to a need for social approval is *heightened sensitivity to social rules and norms*. Here, we see in clients with IBS some very high standards of behavior for themselves and others. They often adhere rigidly to ideas about what is appropriate or inappropriate, responsible or irresponsible. This theme is exemplified by L. M., a 38-year-old female nursing supervisor, who experiences terrible abdominal cramps when she feels she may not make it into work on time, even if she will only be late by a few minutes, and even if there is a reasonable explanation for her tardiness. She gets incensed when any of her staff are late and accepts no excuses, claiming that any responsible person would anticipate potential problems. When she is late herself, she makes sure to work overtime to compensate for time lost, and she expects the same from the other nurses.

Another theme in the experiences of clients with IBS is *perfectionism*. This theme is most commonly represented by the very high standards these clients have for themselves, so that there is little flexibility for failure or flaws. The case of D. E. illustrates this well. D. E., a 40-year-old male business executive, had been in therapy to help him manage and cope with his IBS symptoms. Among other things, treatment had focused on the various stressors in his life and how his symptoms were associated with his level of stress. D. E. had made gains in identifying his stressors and trying out new ways of managing his stress, which helped alleviate some of his symptoms. Still, he had not eradicated either the stress or the symptoms from his life; therefore, he considered therapy to be a failure. His lack of "complete success," defined by him as the total absence of stress and symptoms, was difficult to accept and led to his feeling discouraged and inadequate.

The theme of *anger/frustration* refers to the sense of anger clients often feel about having to cope with a functional bowel disorder, and their frustration with the symptoms themselves. One 22-year-old female client, E. F., a law student, provides an illustration of this theme. Her experience was that life had dealt her an unfair blow in saddling her with IBS, and she was angry that she would have to cope with her bowel problems while other people were able to live their lives without having to pay such attention to their bodily functions. E. F. was not only mad about having IBS, but she spoke of how the symptoms, and her worry about them, interfered with her experience at school and her concentration on her studies.

Another theme, that of *pain*, refers to the fact that many clients with IBS have to cope with symptoms that are often highly painful. One female client, a 40-year-old woman named F. G., speaks of having difficulty taking care of her two young children each day while she often experiences terrible abdominal pain. Her pain makes it impossible for her to be playful with her children in the way she would like, and very often, she spends her time at home lying in bed while they play by themselves.

A theme of *self-efficacy* should be explored. This is characterized by clients with IBS feeling that they are unable to cope with their bowel symptoms. I. J., a 50-year-old female store clerk, expresses a lack of confidence in her abilities to manage her symptoms sufficiently to continue working. Although she considers herself to be a resilient person, having to cope with her chronic diarrhea and abdominal pain leaves her feeling emotionally and physically exhausted, and she is now unsure whether she is strong enough to deal with her IBS.

Next is the theme of *embarrassment/shame*. Clients with IBS commonly express extreme embarrassment about the nature of their physical ailment, given that it is one for which there is no known cause or cure, as well as the fact that symptoms often demand frequent bathroom visits and restricted eating. J. K., a 35-year-old male accountant, has been reluctant to enter into a romantic relationship for fear that once any woman found out about his IBS, she would want to end the relationship. He says that he would not have this concern if he had a disease such as diabetes, or asthma, but he believes that no woman would want to be with a man who "can't even control his bowels."

The final theme is that of *self-nurturance*, which speaks to the experience of many clients with IBS in that they have difficulty taking their own needs and wants into consideration, putting others' concerns ahead of their own. For M. N., a woman in her mid-forties, this theme plays a prominent role in her experience. She speaks about how different it is for her to be in therapy, talking about herself, and how, although she is enjoying it, she feels guilty about taking up this time for herself. She continued to explain how she has never focused solely on herself, so that this was a foreign experience for her, and how she had always been the kind of person people rely on for support, whether friends, family, or colleagues. Throughout her therapy, this woman struggled with taking pleasure in focusing on herself, and felt guilty about doing this very "selfish" work.

Similarly, coping styles may contribute to more or less effective responses to symptoms. The relative degree of "engaged" (e.g., support or information seeking) versus "disengaged" (e.g., escape–avoidance) coping styles may be assessed by the Ways of Coping Inventory (Lazarus & Folkman, 1984). Treatment may often involve encouraging the client to embark on more engaged styles of coping, such as empirically testing limits to activities or levels of anticipated discomfort in various settings, or actively disputing unhelpful thinking patterns.

Some individuals may have learned patterns of illness behavior from early experiences or from observing family members react to physical illness. The therapist should determine whether there is a past history of significant illness for the client or among family members.

Appropriateness for Cognitive-Behavioral Therapy

Cognitive-behavioral therapy is most effective for those who are verbally articulate and capable of psychological insight, although individuals with limited education and psychological sophistication may also profit substantially from this approach. Perhaps the most critical aspect of assessing clients for their appropriateness for a cognitive-behavioral approach is their ability to access automatic thoughts. Some individuals have great difficulty in tuning in to their interior monologues and appear to experience psychological distress almost exclusively in physical symptoms.

Commitment to a cognitive-behavioral treatment approach is important due to clients' investment of the time and effort necessary for improvement. During the initial sessions when the cognitive-behavioral model is being introduced, the therapist should determine how accepting the client is of this approach.

Appropriateness for Group Treatment

During the assessment, the therapist and client should determine whether group or individual therapy is most appropriate. Clients with IBS can derive major benefit from a group setting as they learn that other people experience the same difficulties as they do. The pervasive sense of stigma that most IBS sufferers experience can be significantly diminished. They also learn vicariously about the strategies that others have found useful in dealing with IBS. Counterindications for inclusion in a group setting would be indicated if an individual were hostile or aggressive to the extent that group functioning might be disrupted, or if there were a high likelihood that serious symptoms of anxiety or panic would interfere with the individual's ability to participate in the group.

Mixed-Sex versus Same-Sex Groups

Cognitive-behavioral therapy in a group setting can be a cost-effective method of delivering treatment, and a group setting may serve to normalize and reduce the stigma of IBS. The literature suggests that more women may experience IBS than men. Clinicians working in areas affecting women, such as infertility or sexual abuse, often endorse a same-sex model for group work, noting that women may be more willing to disclose shame-related issues with other women than in a mixed-sex group. On the other hand, the IBS groups conducted in the Toner et al. (1998) study adopted a mixed-sex group format, and a majority of participants indicated that they preferred the mixed-sex setting, noting that this format more closely resembled real life. However, issues of sexual, physical, and emotional abuse, which subsequent research had documented, would probably be much more difficult to discuss in mixed-sex groups.

5

Cognitive-Behavioral
Group Therapy for IBS:
Overview and Initial Session

Overview of Treatment Protocol

The treatment protocol used by our group begins with an initial individual session followed by 12 weekly group sessions, each running 90 minutes. The group is closed-ended; that is, all members start and finish treatment at the same time. As noted earlier, our research was done with groups of six, but we feel groups of four to eight members, plus therapist, can also work well. A second individual session is held after the sixth group session. Its purpose is to review the individual's progress and to clarify any issues regarding the group.

The purposes of the initial individual session are to establish initial rapport with the client, to identify treatment goals, and to begin teaching clients about the theoretical and therapeutic rationale for cognitive-behavioral therapy. In particular, the cognitive-behavioral model is used to highlight how certain cognitions and underlying beliefs may lead to increased attention to bodily sensations, increased arousal, heightened sensitivity to pain, and other IBS symptoms. The model takes into account how IBS

symptoms may become perpetuated by an interplay among biological, psychological, and social factors.

Each of the 12 group sessions follows a standard format with a
predetermined agenda. At the center of each group session is the
introduction of a specific IBS-relevant theme. Our treatment protocol is structured to introduce basic cognitive-behavioral concepts and skills during the initial group sessions together with the
key themes. Subsequent sessions introduce specific IBS-related
coping themes. Specific cognitive-behavioral skills and concepts
introduced in initial sessions include relaxation techniques, techniques for coping with pain, identification of automatic thoughts,
self-monitoring techniques, identification of problem thinking
patterns, techniques for disputing automatic thoughts and negative thinking patterns, and techniques for testing negative beliefs.
In later sessions, these cognitive-behavioral techniques are applied
to specific IBS-related themes. We strongly recommend that the
first three issues discussed be the basic cognitive-behavioral concepts and techniques, pain management, and bowel performance
anxiety. The inclusion and sequencing of the other issues can be
changed to fit the needs of the particular group. These other issues
are shame, anger and assertion, self-efficacy, social approval and
perfectionism, and control.

An overview of a sample course of treatment, based on the
sequence in our protocol, might look as follows:

Pretreatment assessment
Session 1: Individual session—Rationale for cognitive-
    behavioral therapy, identification of individual treat-
    ment goals.
Session 2: Group session theme—Association among
    thoughts, feelings, behavior, and bowel symptoms,
    Part 1.
Session 3: Group session theme—Association among
    thoughts, feelings, behavior, and bowel symptoms,
    Part 2.
Session 4: Group session theme—Pain management.
Session 5: Group session theme—Bowel performance
    anxiety.
Session 6: Group session theme—Shame.

Session 7: Group session theme—Anger and assertion.
Session 8: Individual session—Evaluate individual's progress in group.
Session 9: Group session theme—Self-efficacy.
Session 10: Group session theme—Social approval and perfectionism.
Session 11: Group session theme—Control.
Session 12: Group session theme—Tailored to group needs.
Session 13: Group session theme—Tailored to group needs.
Session 14: Group session theme—Termination.

Standard Group Session Format

Each of the group sessions follows a standard format, which includes the following:

1. Practice progressive relaxation exercise to begin the session (5–10 minutes).
2. Ask for clients' reactions to the previous session (5 minutes). Clients' thoughts and feelings about the previous session serve to keep tabs on the progress of therapy and to clarify any issues about technique or theory introduced during the previous sessions. This process also serves to identify any problems or ruptures in the therapeutic alliance interfering with progress.
3. Review clients' self-help assignments and significant events during the week (15–20 minutes). Review of self-help assignments (e.g., automatic thought records or behavioral experiments) serves to track participants' progress in implementing cognitive skills in situations outside of the group session. Symptom diaries are collected and reviewed as part of this process, with the specific goal of linking stressful events with symptoms. As well as being an opportunity for individual coaching from the therapist, this process serves as an important opportunity for vicarious learning for group members and a positive, success-focused atmosphere in the group. During this checkup process, individual agenda items from participants' reports of relevant personal events are garnered. These can provide a focus for group discussion and exploration.

It is important to monitor progress toward therapy goals and to ensure that self-help assignments are being completed or attempted. Concurrent monitoring of mood (whether formal or informal) serves to reinforce the link between behavior and emotion, and when clients' sense of mastery increases as assignments provide the evidence of progress or new learning, motivation is increased. Decreases in mood or failures to successfully complete assignments show where therapeutic attention is needed.

4. Introduce the session theme (15–20 minutes). Our treatment protocol is structured to introduce and practice cognitive skills during the initial sessions, while subsequent sessions include discussion of specific themes related to IBS, such as shame, bowel performance anxiety, anger and assertion, self-efficacy, social approval, perfectionism, and control. This part of the session includes both a didactic overview of the skill or theme and discussion of the relevance of the theme to the specific concerns of group members. Often these themes are accompanied by handouts for group members, which they can take home to reread.

5. Discuss selected individual agenda items (20–30 minutes). Agenda items are selected collaboratively between therapist and participant based on the material brought forward during the checkup or during group discussion of themes. The focus of the discussion of individual agenda items is on those aspects of clients' experience associated with high negative affect, since schema-based responses tend to emerge specifically in the presence of high affect. These experiences are often brought up by self-help experiments, since such assignments typically are selected on the basis of their likelihood of evoking anxiety. It is during this part of the session that the bulk of therapy occurs. This phase of the group usually takes 20–30 minutes.

6. Give new self-help assignments (10 minutes). Clients are asked to collect evidence about various aspects of current or proposed alternative belief systems. This evidence serves as the basis of subsequent therapeutic exploration. It is an important component to a cognitive-behavioral approach.

7. Summarize session (5 minutes). The purpose of a summary of the session is to reinforce learning, highlight emergent issues, and support achievements. It also serves to reinforce the collaborative nature of the process by giving clients an opportu-

nity to compare their perceptions of the session with the therapist's and with each other.

8. Ask participants' reaction to current session (5 minutes). This gives clients the opportunity to correct any possible miscommunications, to clarify points of confusion, and to flag any problems or ruptures in the therapeutic alliance in a timely manner.

The Initial Individual Session

As mentioned earlier, the main tasks to be accomplished in the initial, individual session are the following:

- Give clients the rationale for cognitive-behavioral therapy.
- Establish initial rapport and a collaborative relationship.
- Identify the individual's treatment goals.
- Introduce relaxation training.

The Importance of a Rationale for Psychotherapeutic Intervention

Not unsurprisingly for people with obvious physical symptoms and pain, people with IBS may interpret referrals to psychologists or psychiatrists as insulting and personally diminishing. The critical challenge to the therapist is to openly address and dispute the idea that IBS symptoms are imaginary or caused by underlying mental problems. Only when this task is successfully addressed is a therapeutic alliance possible.

The main task of the therapist, therefore, in the initial session with the client with IBS and throughout therapy is to present a rationale for cognitive-behavioral intervention that recognizes the tangible reality of IBS symptoms, while suggesting a role for cognitive-behavioral techniques in reducing or alleviating those symptoms. The essence of this approach is to give equal weight to physical stressors (fatigue, spicy food, illness) and psychosocial stressors (being late, feeling self-conscious, being angry) that may trigger IBS symptoms. The second task of the therapist is to establish a collaborative relationship by explaining the need for clients to take an active role.

Validating the Reality of Physical Symptoms

Therapists needs to convey the message that they know the client's pain is real, and that they have confidence the procedures used in cognitive-behavioral therapy will be beneficial. The therapist may also suggest to the client that "I am not asking you to believe me on faith, but rather encouraging you to work with me. If you are willing to give it a try, I believe you will be surprised to learn how much control you can have over your IBS symptoms" (Holzman & Turk, 1986).

It is critical to solicit questions. Many clients with IBS tend to be unassertive in therapists' offices. For clients who do not ask questions, it is often worthwhile to say something such as, "Although it may not have occurred to you yet, many clients are often concerned about. . . . " These concerns may focus on the belief that because we are mental health professionals, only people with imaginary IBS symptoms get referred, or that we will not take their IBS symptoms seriously. It is likely the client is thinking about these things; if not addressed, these fears and concerns may interfere with their participation in therapy (Holzman & Turk, 1986). We found that the therapeutic alliance is enhanced by validating the reality of symptoms and also challenging society's view of the artificial dualism of functional/organic components of illness. For example, the health care provider might want to address the dualism directly with the client during an initial visit. The following is an example of how the therapist might describe this artificial dualism to clients with IBS.

Possible Script for a Rationale

There are many myths about IBS. One such myth is that if physicians cannot yet identify a physical cause, then the symptoms are trivial or unimportant. But this is not true. We know that living with IBS can severely compromise your quality of life. For example, living with chronic and unpredictable pain and diarrhea is not easy and can interfere with work and social activities.

Another myth is that if physicians cannot yet pinpoint a physical problem, then the symptoms must be all in your head. In other words, the symptoms are somehow less real. Again, research has established that this is simply not true. IBS is a real disorder related to heightened gut motility (muscle contraction), sensation, or both. Symptoms can be influenced by a variety of factors such as food, hormones, activity, and stress.

The gut shares many nerve pathways and chemical transmitters with the brain and is sometimes called the little brain. The gut nervous system (or little brain), responds to the brain's input under various conditions. For example, under stress, the brain may send messages to the gut that heighten the sensitivity of the gut nerve receptors. We now know that IBS is not caused by stress but that stress may further aggravate bowel symptoms. We also know that stress can cause bowel symptoms in most people. However, studies have revealed that people with IBS are more reactive since they already have a hypersensitive gut and therefore are likely to experience more symptoms under any type of stress, whether psychological, physical, dietary, or hormonal. Research has also indicated that if persons with IBS also suffer from depression or anxiety, their bowel symptoms may get worse during episodes of depression and anxiety. While there is no effective medication or cure for IBS, we can help you reduce your symptoms and feel better. However, this requires that we have a shared plan of care. You are the best expert in identifying what makes your bowel symptoms better.

The therapist should also be aware of the fact that in spite of our growing understanding of IBS, there are additional myths associated with it that persist. Here is a brief discussion of a sampling of such myths.

1. *IBS is a psychiatric disorder.* This myth persists for a number of reasons. Since antidepressants have been known to be used in the treatment of IBS, some people feel IBS is simply some form of depression. It is important to highlight the rationale for the administration of antidepressants for IBS. To begin with, antidepressants act in doses lower than that prescribed for depression on certain areas of the brain to release chemicals (neurotransmitters) that block pain. In addition to the treatment of IBS, antidepressants have been known to be effective in other medical conditions including headaches and diabetic pain. An-

other reason why this myth persists is that people who present with IBS to gastroenterologists and take part in studies may also meet criteria for an associated anxiety or a depressive disorder. Studies have found that about half of the people who are seen in gastroenterology clinics with IBS may also meet criteria for anxiety and/or depression. There are many possible explanations for this association including: (1) anxiety and depression, like IBS, are common in the general population, especially among women, so their co-occurrence may be simply due to this high frequency; (2) we know that people who may also have an associated anxiety or depressive disorder may be having more difficulty coping with the IBS symptoms and seek specialized help for their IBS at higher rates than people with IBS who might not have an associated anxiety or depressive disorder; and (3) depression and anxiety may be a consequence of living with a chronic, debilitating disorder such as IBS.

2. *If pain is severe, there must be an organic cause.* This common myth persists as a function of our Western society's false conceptualization of pain (i.e., if the pain is severe, there must be a structural cause). The experience of pain is a consequence of a complex interaction among physical, cognitive, emotional and behavioral components. The gate theory of pain helps explain this multifactorial event. It states that pain messages originate at the site of the bodily damage, injury, or disease and are then passed through a mechanism that works like a gate to the brain. The brain then interprets the pain message, and it is at this point the pain is experienced. The pain gate can be partially or fully opened or closed, determining the amount of pain experienced. Factors that can open the gate (i.e., those that make the pain more central or more intense) include thoughts that focus attention on the pain. Feelings that can open the gate include depression, anxiety, and anger. Behaviors can also open the gate, such as lack of pleasant activities. Factors that can close the gate (i.e., those that make the pain less central or less intense) include coping strategies such as controlling pain thoughts through attention diversion. Examples of attention diversion are distraction, imagery, and relaxation. Cognitive strategies such as altering the self-talk to messages such as "I can handle this, I handled this before" versus "I can't stand another second of this pain" are also useful in reducing the intensity of the pain.

3. *Clients with IBS may "benefit" from the "sick role."* This myth has pejorative connotations and is an unhelpful formulation for health care providers and clients. Myths persist based on a traditional notion in psychiatry that some clients achieve some gain or benefit through their illness. People with IBS do not want to be ill and do not take any pleasure from this chronic and debilitating illness. It is true that having a chronic illness may result in a person receiving more attention from others, being released from some usual responsibilities, and having social and financial compensation. However, it is important to note that there is no empirical support to validate the notion that clients seek out or wish to benefit from living with IBS. Rather, clients with IBS are interested in overcoming this painful disorder that reduces their quality of life.

4. *People with IBS are difficult clients.* Again, this myth is not true. Rather, IBS is a difficult disorder associated with little information and a great deal of stigma and trivialization. The lack of information, coupled with the shame and trivialization associated with having not only a so-called "psychosomatic" or "functional" disorder, but also a disorder involving the bowels, leads to frustration and further distress in clients. Since most health care professionals including physicians are not adequately trained in the conceptualization and/or treatment of IBS, this may elicit uncomfortable feelings from them, which may lead some health care providers to feel helpless in treating IBS. It is important to recognize, from both the client's and the health care provider's point of view, that this is a frustrating disorder with many unanswered questions. An honest and open discussion acknowledging the frustrations associated with this disorder would be helpful. It is important for both the client and health care provider to work in a collaborative fashion to try to understand what will be most helpful to manage the symptoms. Since there is no effective medication or cure for IBS, the focus needs to be directed at symptom management and coping with this chronic condition. However, improved symptom control requires a shared plan of care between the health care professional and the client. Treatment plans tailored to clients' individual needs and concerns will ensure that those with IBS can cope with their conditions as comfortably as possible and with minimal disruption to everyday life.

Establishing a Collaborative Relationship:
The Client as a Personal Scientist

This initial session begins the collaborative process that will be critical in subsequent sessions. As previously mentioned, inherent in all the cognitive-behavioral therapies is the notion that the client is the "expert" related to his/her own situation. Questions are phrased in a manner requiring judgment on the part of the client and respect for his/her beliefs. The therapist does not generally assume the role of the expert, but rather assumes the role of the facilitator. This approach establishes the collaborative relationship that is central to the cognitive-behavioral intervention (cf. Turk et al., 1978; Holzman & Turk, 1986).

Clients need to be informed that they are the best people to evaluate their own experience. In order to help them do this, we invite them to collaborate with us in a manner similar to the way a scientist evaluates data he/she has gathered to see whether the facts fit the theories. Theories that clients with IBS may have about their functioning (e.g., that they are victims of their diseases, they have no control over their bodily reactions, or that stress is something that happens to them from the outside, over which they have little control) can then be evaluated in the open. An attempt to encourage clients to be personal scientists involves three steps. The first of these is to encourage them to gather information about their thoughts and emotions in stressful situations. The second step involves asking them to examine whether there is any relationship between these pieces of information. Therapists can be particularly helpful in this phase by pointing out possible connections between thoughts and feelings. The third step involves helping clients to become aware of the hypotheses they have and to examine whether the data they collect support or do not support those hypotheses.

An example here might be a client who believes that a need for emotional contact with others or overt displays of affection are signs of weakness. The client can be asked to consider this belief as a theory that may or may not be supported.

Gathering information about the theory's support may involve asking other people how they feel about the expression of emotion, examining the patterns of emotional expression in the family, or recalling instances in which the client felt good about other people expressing emotion to him/her. In this way, this disconfirmatory evidence has a chance to compete with the usual information clients give themselves and perhaps challenge some of their unhelpful attitudes about relating to others.

The value of this stance for the therapist is that he/she avoids the trap of being in a position to tell clients that he/she knows what is best for them. At the same time, however, the therapist can reassure the client that this process has been found to be helpful in the past, and that there is good reason to believe that it will continue to be so in their case. This, therefore, allows the therapist to increase client expectancies for change, while at the same time avoiding an unnecessarily optimistic stance regarding the client's condition, which some clients may utilize as further reason for disproving the therapist and confirming their own sense of demoralization.

Understanding IBS in Cognitive-Behavioral Terms

An initial task of the collaborative process is to develop a personalized model of the impact of the bowel disorder for the client, using a cognitive-behavioral framework. Such a model reflects the client's perception of the nature of the symptoms. Four aspects of the client's environment are interconnected and each influences all of the others (Padesky & Greenberger, 1995). These elements include thoughts (beliefs, images, memories), moods, behaviors, and physical reactions, all of which take place in the client's social context (past and present). Each aspect of life influences all the others, and small changes in one area can lead to changes in other areas. For example, changes in behavior influence how we think and how we feel. To illustrate this model, suppose a client reports that her abdominal pain worries her because she fears that she has undiagnosed cancer, or because her symptoms prevent her from fulfilling her family obligations. The therapist may find it useful to draw a schematic diagram, like that presented in Figure 5.1, to channel the client's description of her situation along cognitive-behavioral lines.

In seeking to assess these aspects of an individual's circum-

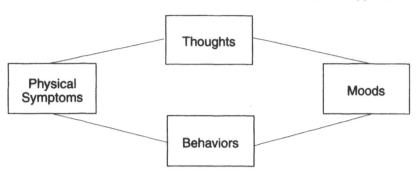

FIGURE 5.1. Social context.

stances, Padesky and Greenberger have outlined a number of questions that the therapist may find useful to explore. These include the following:

1. *Environmental changes/social context:* Has the client experienced any recent changes? What have been the most stressful events during the past year? Three years? Five years? In childhood? Are there any long-term or ongoing difficulties (such as discrimination or harassment by others)? How do socialized role expectations and power imbalances permeate the person's life?

2. *Physical reactions:* Are there any troubling physical symptoms such as changes in energy level, appetite, or sleep? What are the specific IBS symptoms, and are there other symptoms, such as sweating or rapid heart rate, that are not specific to IBS?

3. *Moods:* What single words describe moods (happy, sad, nervous, ashamed)? How are moods affected by symptoms? Is the primary mood depression? Frustration? Anxiety?

4. *Behaviors:* What specific behaviors would the client like to change or improve? At home? At work? With friends? Alone? Does the client avoid situations or people when it might be of benefit to be involved?

5. *Thoughts:* When there are strong moods, what are the accompanying thoughts about the self? Other people? The

future? What thoughts interfere with things that would be pleasant or productive to do? Do any images or memories accompany these thoughts?

These questions serve to outline the salient components that affect a client's experience of IBS. It is useful to understand in general terms the nature of each of these factors before proceeding to the specific formulation.

FORMULATION OF THE CLIENT'S IBS IN COGNITIVE-BEHAVIORAL TERMS

In developing a formulation at the initial session with a client, the method described by Salkovskis (1992) is useful. Salkovskis notes that the central issue in somatic disorders is the negative thinking and anxious focusing on perceived threat. Of particular relevance is not the actual probability of the perceived threat, but the perceived cost of the threat. In other words, although the probability of the threat may be low, there is an "awfulness" about the threat that escalates anxiety. Therefore, it is not always useful to dispute rationally the probability of a feared outcome. In fact, Salkovskis notes that reassurance, in and of itself, is typically unhelpful, if not counterproductive.

Salkovskis (1995) describes a formulation technique, which is illustrated in Figure 5.2. For any specified event or episode, there may be a trigger event (going for a long car ride, attending a meeting) that initiates an episode of bowel distress. The components to the episodes are identification of a perceived threat, feelings of apprehension or anxiety, awareness of bodily sensations such as pain or urgency, and interpretations of the bodily sensations as catastrophic ("I'll have an accident"). These components act to potentiate and reinforce each other, so that as apprehension increases, bodily sensations become more noticeable, and interpretations of sensations become more threatening. The upward spiral of cognitions, sensations, and emotions is rapid, sometimes occurring in seconds, and may not be easily separable into their components by the client.

In developing the formulation with the client, the therapist

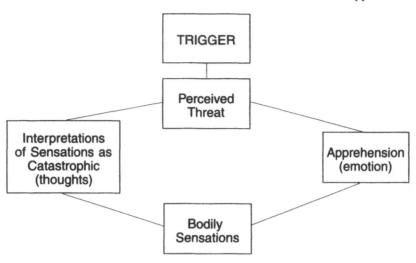

FIGURE 5.2. Relationship among threats, apprehension, and symptoms.

selects a recent, specific incident or episode that was relatively severe. This may be when pain was intense, when diarrhea was severe, or when the client feared that she would lose control of her
bowels. The therapist should constantly re-refer to this incident
("At that time, . . . ") when questioning the client, so as to maintain a specific focus on that incident. Throughout the course of
developing the formulation, the therapist should use frequent
feedback and summaries of all that has gone before, sequentially
building up the picture of the client's subjective experience and
its sequence in the client's mind.

The formulation should begin with whatever point the client first addresses, whether that be feelings of anxiety, bodily
sensations, or cognitions. The sequence to follow, regardless of
where it is entered, is sensation–thoughts–emotions–sensation–
thoughts, and so on. The therapist should pinpoint the moment
when the anxiety or distress was worse, and proceed from that
point.

Questions that the therapist may use in developing the formulation include the following: "What was going through your
mind right at that moment?", with a follow-up of "At that time,
what did you think was the worst thing that could happen?", fol-

lowed by "When you had that thought, how did that make you feel?", "When you began to feel that emotion, what symptoms did you notice?", and "When you noticed those symptoms increased, what went through your mind?" These questions should aid in specifying the specific thoughts, feelings, and symptoms that characterize a client's distress.

SETTING GOALS AND DISCUSSING PERFECTIONISM

Once an initial formulation has been developed, the collaborative process is continued through the establishment of goals for therapy. Goal setting typically is initiated in the first session. Similar to the contract in any therapeutic relationship, Holzman and Turk (1986) feel that the formal establishment of observable, measurable, and mutually agreed-upon goals is essential for treatment progress and for avoiding missed communications and inappropriate expectations. Therapy goals are individually negotiated and are thus unique for each client. They are developed in consideration of the individual's current status, his/her particular strengths and challenges, and the more general goals for treatment. The result of the negotiation process must be the establishment of goals that the individual feels are obtainable as well as personally relevant to his/her particular needs. Thus, individualized treatment goals cannot be dictated to the client. They must be individually considered and emanate from the client's needs. Discussion of the common themes that are relevant to individuals who present with IBS (e.g., pain management, need for approval, unassertiveness, perfectionistic beliefs, "bowel performance" anxiety, anger, control) may help elicit client needs and set the stage for the elaboration of personal goals in therapy.

Clients often come to the cognitive-behavioral therapy group with the belief that therapy will abolish their symptoms. It is important to emphasize that the goals of the cognitive-behavioral intervention are to provide clients with new skills to identify stress and helpful coping strategies to deal with their IBS symptoms rather that to "cure IBS." Despite such explanation, many individuals with IBS have very perfectionistic beliefs regarding therapy. The perfectionistic beliefs can interfere with clients' maintaining new skills and ways of coping. For example, clients may believe that by the end of therapy "I won't be hindered by my IBS symptoms or won't have symptoms." But such clients are likely to experience increased levels of anxiety as the end of therapy approaches and they realize that therapy is falling short of their expectations. It is important at the start of treatment to explore perfectionistic views of outcome. Such clients may decide that unless the new ways of coping cure, they should be abandoned.

INTRODUCTION OF RELAXATION TRAINING

Relaxation training with 16 muscle groups (adapted from Bernstein & Borkovec, 1973) is offered to clients in this cognitive-behavioral treatment package as a coping skill. We make the point to clients that the connections between cognitions and physical symptoms are reciprocal; not only can changing stress-inducing cognitions reduce physical symptoms, but also damping down bodily tension may lead to increased feelings of well-being and reduced bowel distress. We also point out that some individuals are so chronically tense that they forget what it feels like to be relaxed. As they practice being physically relaxed, they become more able to differentiate between tense and relaxed states. Sometimes clients discover through this process that they are indeed chronically tense, and are in fact using their "gut responses" to guide their behavior. Though relaxation techniques, clients learn new methods for attaining physical calmness and increase their sense that symptoms can be controlled.

The basic procedures of relaxation training involve moving the focus by tensing and untensing various muscle groups throughout the body. These are generally located in the hands, the head, moving to the chest, shoulders, and torso area, then down to the thigh, calf, and foot areas. Clients sit comfortably in their chairs while the therapist reviews the rationale and explains the relaxation technique. In the basic procedure, clients are asked to make a tight fist or tense the muscle in that area to notice what that tension or feeling is like and then to release and be psychologically aware of the contrast between the two feeling states, with the second state being labeled relaxation and the first labeled tension.

Most of the points made during the initial session are repeated many times in treatment. Therefore, these issues are not critical for the client to recall. What is most important is that the client leave with a general understanding and positive attitude toward the program, a general willingness to actively participate, and an expectation for treatment success (Holzman & Turk, 1986).

6

Key Themes and Skills
in the Treatment of IBS

The initial individual session introduces members to the basic rationale for cognitive-behavioral treatment of IBS. The first group sessions begin applying that model to the specific experiences of group members. We strongly recommend that these first group sessions introduce key cognitive concepts and skills as well as give priority to the issues of pain management and bowel performance anxiety. The inclusion or ordering of the other issues can be adapted to the goals and emerging issues of a given group.

In the balance of this chapter, we detail the specific new content and skills to be introduced in the first three to four group sessions. Table 6.1 summarizes the standard group session format described in Chapter 5. Note that each new content area in this and following chapters represents only one section (item 4 in Table 6.1) within the larger session format. We start with the initial two group sessions that focus on the association among thoughts, feelings, behavior, and bowel symptoms.

TABLE 6.1. Standard Group Session Format

1. Begin with relaxation exercise (5–10 minutes).
2. Ask for clients' reactions to previous session (for first group session, this would be the previous individual session) (5 minutes).
3. Review self-help assignments (except for the first group session, where there have not yet been assignments) (15–20 minutes).
4. Introduce session theme and related skills (15–20 minutes).[a]
5. Discuss selected individual agenda items (20–30 minutes).
6. Select new self-help assignments (10 minutes).
7. Summarize session (5 minutes).
8. Ask for clients' reactions to current session (5 minutes).

[a]See Chapters 6, 7, and 8 for specific content by session theme.

Session Theme: Association among Thoughts, Feelings, Behavior, and Bowel Symptoms

The major focus of cognitive-behavioral therapy is the systematic evaluation of the perceptions, thoughts, belief systems, and assumptions that underlie behavior and are connected closely to mood. The first step in this process is to identify the specific patterns of thinking that are associated with IBS, associated behaviors, and moods.

For example, an individual with IBS may experience some bothersome bowel symptoms during a period of illness or environmental stress. If these symptoms are potentially embarrassing, such as excessive gas or bowel urgency, the person may develop certain beliefs that interfere with spontaneous behaviors. For example, he/she may come to believe that certain social events or situations are not "safe" because there is not a bathroom easily available. The individual may then become reluctant to engage in social events away from home and avoid or escape from such situations. This pattern of behavior can make an individual feel depressed, anxious, or angry. These feelings in themselves contribute to physiological arousal and increase the likelihood and severity of bowel symptoms.

Each of these factors contributes to and influences the others. For example, if a person believes she is "safe" at home, she will not be as anxious, her physical arousal will be less, and her symptoms will likely be less bothersome than if she were out at a public function. The role of the thought here is central. For example, if something happens that changes the "safe" situation to a "threatening" one, such as the arrival of an unfamiliar visitor, it is likely that the mood of calm would change to anxiety and bowel symptoms might rapidly appear. The evaluation of the situation as "safe" or "threatening" is the major predictor of the person's mood and physical symptoms.

Given the critical role of the evaluation and interpretation of the situation, cognitive-behavioral therapy encourages clients to pay attention to the specific cognitions associated with their bowel symptoms. This is often a new approach for individuals who have focused almost exclusively on the biological factors affecting their symptoms. Once the links between cognitions, moods, behaviors, and symptoms are made, the next task of therapy is to identify unhelpful patterns of thinking that shape perceptions and lead to unhelpful behaviors. Then the therapist assists the client in practicing alternative patterns of thinking through cognitive restructuring techniques, such as helpful responses.

We have found it helpful to introduce this content in two parts, over two group sessions.

Session Theme: Association of Thoughts, Feelings, Behavior, and Bowel Symptoms, Part 1

Points to cover

- Validate reality of physical and environmental stressors.
- Explain three major parts of stress reactions: the physical, the behavioral, and the cognitive.
- Discuss how events and their appraisal lead to emotional reactions.
- Introduce and discuss how to identify automatic thoughts.
- Introduce Daily Thought Record (first three columns).

In the initial individual session, the therapist presents a brief rationale for cognitive-behavioral therapy to the client. Together they then develop a formulation of the client's IBS that includes thoughts, feelings, behavior, and bowel symptoms. In the first group session, the therapist reviews the association among thoughts, feelings, behavior, and bowel symptoms and helps clients begin to see it at work in their own situations. Clients' formulations can serve as salient examples throughout the discussion.

The following discussion may be helpful in integrating cognitive components to the client's own theoretical model of his/her bowel difficulties. As with the initial individual session, however, it is helpful to begin with validation of the physical symptoms.

The following is a possible script that therapists might follow in order to relate the cognitive-behavioral approach to bowel disorders.

Biological Vulnerabilities

We are all born with certain biological strengths and weaknesses. Some of our organ systems are stronger or weaker than others. As we get older, some of us will develop heart disease, diabetes, or back problems. It is likely that we have some biological predisposition to develop physical problems, and when we review our family history, we may learn that our grandmother had diabetes or that everyone on our father's side of the family has a bad right knee.

Environmental Stressors

In addition to a biological or genetic basis for physical problems, sometimes aspects of the environment may bring on a specific symptom. For example, for the person with a family history of heart disease, eating a high-fat diet and smoking can result in heart problems, while the same behavior causes no symptoms for someone without a family history of heart trouble. Similarly, a viral illness can result in the onset of certain autoimmune disorders, such as rheumatoid arthritis, in some affected individuals but not in others.

It is likely that IBS is due to a similar interaction between biological tendencies and environmental stressors. Environmental factors may include illnesses or medical treatments that disrupt normal bowel functioning, food allergies or sensitivities, or stressful life events that result in acute or chronic states of arousal. If an individual has a biological vulnerability to gastrointestinal disorders (e.g., hypersensitive gut, enhanced motility and visceral sensation), these environmental factors can "tip them over the edge," resulting in chronic bowel problems.

There are numerous factors that may influence the onset of IBS. They may be short-term events, such as drinking coffee, or more long-term causes, such as a "triggering" illness that may have made the bowel hypersensitive. Which factors can you identify that may have triggered bowel symptoms for you?

Categories may include lack of sleep, certain foods (milk, spicy foods, coffee, alcohol), temporary illnesses (flu), weather (heat, barometric changes), having a high-stress job, traveling (jet lag), a genetic predisposition to irritable bowel, medications, and family arguments or disputes at work. [Clients should be encouraged to come up with a range of triggers, while the therapist points out that every person has different triggers.]

It is apparent that any number of triggers can result in symptoms. Some triggers are physical stressors. Some are psychological stressors. Some are short-term; others are long-term. They are similar in that they all cause a stress response that includes bowel symptoms.

What Is a Stress Response?

A stress response is an arousal of the autonomic nervous system. This arousal includes a set of predictable physical events. The brain releases stress hormones and our bodies prepare for "fight or flight." The heart rate speeds up to supply blood to the large muscle groups, the breathing gets faster to increase the oxygen supply, and the liver releases glucose to provide fuel for the muscles. The blood supply is diverted from the gut to the large muscles to enable the body to fight or flee. The results of this diversion are a slowing of gut motility and sometimes an urge to void or defecate. The body is getting the message that it has more important things to do than digest or eliminate.

Although a number of the listed factors causing stress are physical (such as drinking coffee or eating spicy foods), some of the stresses we encounter are psychosocial, such as a high-stress job or a traffic jam. Regardless of whether the stressor is physical or psychosocial, the reaction is exactly the same: arousal resulting in symptoms.

Although these body reactions occur as a result of a "trigger" or short-term stress, in many cases, stress goes on for long periods of time, resulting in a state of chronic, recurring arousal. During long-term stress, the gut is deluged with messages to slow down or speed up, and after a while, the regulating mechanisms of bowel function are unable to perform the fine adjustments necessary for normal functioning. The gut may become hypersensitive, reacting to low levels of stimulation with severe reactions.

The Three Components of Stress

Stress has three major parts: the physical, the behavioral, and the cognitive. Although everyone experiences these factors differently, there are usually common elements to our experience of each of these aspects of stress.

Physical symptoms of stress include all of the bowel symptoms that we have described. If arousal from stress continues over a long period of time with no relief, we may become exhausted. Every activity becomes an effort and we lose our motivation to start new tasks or to fulfill our obligations. As time passes, sleep, appetite, and sex drive may be disrupted, and we may become depressed or anxious.

Behavioral symptoms of stress are varied. They include how you act and what you do because of the stress. For example, you can spend a lot of time learning the location of washrooms or you might avoid or withdraw from situations you used to enjoy, such as eating in restaurants. Other behavioral symptoms of stress may include irritability, restlessness, or overuse of alcohol or medications.

The cognitive aspects of stress will be the main focus of cognitive-behavioral treatment. By "cognitive" we mean thoughts, beliefs, attitudes, and specific ways of thinking about IBS.

In addition to events that are obviously stressful (slamming on the brakes to avoid an accident), there are situations that become stressful because of the way we think about them. For example, running into an old friend might not be stressful—unless the last time you met this friend you poured tomato juice into her lap. In other words, a neutral or positive event (seeing a friend) is turned into a negative or stressful event because of how we think about the situation.

We bring more than our thoughts to situations; we also bring our attitudes and beliefs. For example, our meeting with an old friend might become stressful if we begin silently to compare our appearance, career success, or level of fitness to our friend's. Even if we feel that we come off well in such comparisons, the belief that friends are making silent criticisms of each other may in itself be an attitude that leads to increased stress.

HOW EVENTS AND THEIR APPRAISAL LEAD
TO EMOTIONAL REACTIONS

This session also tries to convey to clients the idea that the reality of an emotional reaction is something that can be broken down into a number of subcomponents. The theory is proposed that emotional reactions are the product of interactions of events and appraisals that are client-initiated. In this way, the overwhelming psychological plausibility of emotions can be broken down into subcomponents, and these subcomponents can then be examined for their veridicality or adaptiveness. For example, in the midst of feeling upset or rejected by an individual, the psychological experience of rejection tends to overwhelm or block out any alternative views of the situation that may be equally plausible. In this case, the emotion leads to a form of emotional reasoning, in that "If I feel a certain way, then my feeling tells me that the way I see the situation is true." The type of thinking presented in this example is called "emotional reasoning." It occurs when people react on the basis of how they are feeling at the time, on an interpretation of what the event means.

In cases of psychological difficulty, some of these methods may be somewhat less than helpful regarding the event itself. By emphasizing to people that emotions are proceeded by thoughts, and that thoughts are appraisals of situations, clients can begin to examine their emotional experience rather than merely be swept up by it and feel as if they have no control over changing it. Finally, a number of definitions of unhelpful cognitions, such as dichotomous thinking, personalization, overgeneralization, and so on, are offered.

AUTOMATIC THOUGHTS

Following the general discussion of the cognitive-behavioral approach to IBS, the client is introduced to the concept of automatic thoughts and given instructions as to how to identify such thoughts and use of the Thought Record (from Greenberger & Padesky, 1995; see Appendix 2).

Possible Script Introducing Automatic Thoughts

It is usually difficult to pay attention to our interpretations of events, not because they are so rare or fleeting, but because they are so common. It is as if we have a VCR playing in the back of our heads that is always on, and it plays tapes we have heard a thousand times before. Sometimes the tape starts running in response to some event that has just occurred, and sometimes it replays past events. Usually we do not pay much attention to what the tape is saying, but sometimes, when we are not distracted by the events of the day, the tape can be the focus of our attention. This often happens late at night, when we are trying to sleep, and old tapes of various embarrassing or upsetting events start to run, much against our will.

Many people complain of constant, ruminative thoughts that they are unable to control or escape. These thoughts form a background to our everyday activities, like a television tuned to a "negativity channel." Because these thoughts are so ever-present, we call them "automatic thoughts." They are also automatic in the sense that they occur without much effort on our part. In fact, it takes some effort to become aware that they are there and what their actual meaning is.

The Thought Record tries to encourage clients to assess the fluctuations of their emotions and cognitive activity. The first three columns of the Record are presented to the client, who is then asked to rate the situation of concern by describing briefly the emotions that were experienced in that situation and writing down any automatic thoughts that came to mind. In this way, clients will begin to notice that in situations they find problematic or distressing, they may be saying things to themselves that may have a direct influence on their mood. It is important for therapists to treat these as provisional hypotheses and to present them to clients in an open manner, so that clients are encouraged to reach their own conclusions on the degree of association between cognitive activity and emotional distress.

Some clients may need help in identifying automatic thoughts, and the therapist can facilitate the process, as is done in the following example:

CLIENT: I had a problem when I was being driven by some friends to a party, but I really didn't have any automatic thoughts. I just knew I was upset.

THERAPIST: What were you most concerned about in this situation?

CLIENT: I was afraid I couldn't last till we got there, and I'd have to ask them to pull over somewhere.

THERAPIST (*writes*): "I can't last till we get there."

CLIENT: "I'll have to ask them to pull over."

THERAPIST: What could happen?

CLIENT: I probably wouldn't have had an accident, but I might have had to ask them to pull over.

THERAPIST: What would have happened if you asked them to pull over?

CLIENT: They would have thought I was weird. I don't really know these people, and they don't know about my problem.

THERAPIST (*writes*): "They'll think I'm weird." How would they think you're weird?

CLIENT: They would probably think I have emotional problems or something, because there would be no reason to lose control.

THERAPIST (*writes*): "They would think I have emotional problems."

CLIENT: They would think less of me.

THERAPIST (*writes*): "They would think less of me."

THERAPIST: It seems that you had a number of thoughts that were adding to your stress in this situation.

CLIENT: I guess I did.

Session Theme: Association among Thoughts, Feelings, Behavior, and Bowel Symptoms, Part 2

Points to cover

- How to identify problem thinking patterns.
- How to use dispute handles to develop more helpful responses.
- How to use the CALM method of developing helpful responses.

GIVING THE FIRST SELF-HELP ASSIGNMENT

Clients are introduced to the concept of weekly self-help assignments and are encouraged to view such assignments as the compilation of data on their progress throughout the course of therapy.

The importance of completing self-help assignments must be stressed as enabling participants to map their acquired skills in coping with IBS as the therapy progresses.

Possible Script Introducing Self-Help Assignment

Our first task for the coming week will be to pay attention to our automatic thoughts. We will do this by using the Thought Record. Only the first three columns will be used at first. In the first column, an upsetting or anxiety-producing situation will be described. The situation should be described as simply as possible, so that automatic thoughts are not used as situational descriptors. In the second column, the emotions associated with the situation are noted, with the strength of those emotions rated on a scale of 1 to 100. Finally, the automatic thoughts associated with the emotions in that situation are described. Automatic thoughts should be described in simple sentences, and questions should be avoided. In addition, it is vitally important to monitor the frequency and severity of bowel symptoms during your participation. Therefore, as part of your self-help assignment, you are also expected to complete the Functional Bowel Disorders Diary Forms of IBS and turn them in next session.

Emphasize the importance of tracking accurate accounts of clients' symptoms. The tracking of bowel symptoms is the first step in helping clients develop an awareness of the exact fluctuations in symptomatology that they experience and can often be used in sessions as an anchor to compare against the reports of symptoms. Therapists may become aware of tendencies to either amplify the magnitude of distress or, alternatively (and more commonly), minimize the magnitude of distress if clients are trying to present their problems as being of a noninterfering nature.

After introducing automatic thoughts during the first group session, subsequent sessions can introduce cognitive skills, including identifying problem thinking patterns and using dispute handles to develop helpful responses. The concept of problem thinking patterns originally termed "cognitive distortions" by Burns (1981), can then be introduced.

PROBLEM THINKING PATTERNS

Individuals with IBS tend to use certain problem thinking patterns more than others. Specifically, since they endorse highly conventional standards of behavior in themselves and others, and see violations of social norms as disturbing, they tend to catastrophize the results of social disapproval. They typically use "should statements" with unquestioning enthusiasm and are often quite rigid in the standards they set for their behavior and presentation. These standards are often represented in their appearance; individuals who have IBS are usually very well-groomed and conservatively dressed. They tend to be more punctual than other clients, more conscientious about completing self-help assignments. Their tendency to catastrophize about the consequences of negative evaluation by others makes them vulnerable to social disapproval. The ten key "problem thinking patterns" to be discussed are (1) all-or-nothing thinking; (2) overgeneralization; (3) mental filter; (4) disqualifying the positive; (5) jumping to conclusions, including both mind reading and fortune telling; (6) magnification or minimization; (7) emotional reasoning; (8) "should" statements; (9) labeling and mislabeling; and (10) personalization. Table 6.2 contains definitions of problem thinking patterns along with IBS examples. Distributing this information as a handout to clients can be helpful.

Working through the examples of automatic thoughts from self-help assignments for the first session will clarify the application of problem thinking patterns to thoughts.

HELPFUL RESPONSES AND DISPUTE HANDLES

When problem thinking patterns have been identified, the next step is to assist the client to practice new thinking patterns. A first step is challenging the assumption that a negative automatic thought must be true. Clients can learn to do this through formu-

TABLE 6.2. Problem Thinking Patterns

1. *All-or-nothing thinking:* You see things in black or white categories. If your performance falls short of perfect, you see yourself as a failure. All-or-nothing thinking can often be identified by the use of such words as "everyone," "no one," "I can never," or "I always," etc.

    Example: "Everyone else can eat a huge meal and feel fine afterwards. I never can. I always have terrible symptoms."

2. *Overgeneralization:* You see a single event as part of a never-ending pattern.

    Example: "I had to get up and leave the seminar in the middle because of my symptoms. This is the second time in 2 months this has happened. Here we go again—I'll never be able to sit through a long meeting."

3. *Mental filter:* You pick out a single negative detail and dwell on it exclusively, so that your vision of reality becomes darkened, like the drop of ink that discolors the entire beaker of water.

    Example: "When I heard my stomach rumble so noisily during the award ceremony, I thought I'd die! That embarrassment ruined the whole experience for me. I know the person next to me noticed."

4. *Disqualifying the positive:* You reject positive experiences by insisting that they "don't count" for some reason or another. In this way, you can maintain a negative belief that is contradicted by your everyday experiences.

    Example: "My family really seems to appreciate my sense of humor. They might think that I'm witty, but it's only because I feel comfortable around them. Why can't I talk like that with other people?"

5. Jumping to conclusions: You make a negative interpretation, even though there are no definite facts that convincingly support your conclusion.

There are two ways to jump to conclusions:

a. *Mind reading:* You arbitrarily conclude that someone is reacting negatively to you and you don't bother to check it out.

    Example: "I can't tell my friend Carol about my IBS; she's a very fastidious person, and I'm sure that she'd be totally disgusted."

b. *Fortune telling:* You anticipate that things will turn out badly, and you feel convinced that your prediction is already an established fact.

    Example: "I would like to go to lunch with the people at work, but I am sure that I would have to go running to the bathroom at least four times during the meal. What's the point in putting myself in that position?"

6. *Magnification (catastophizing) or minimization:* You exaggerate the importance of things (such as your bowel symptoms, or someone else's social confidence), or you inappropriately shrink things until they appear tiny (your accomplishments or the other person's imperfections). This is called "the binocular trick."

(continued)

TABLE 6.2. *(cont.)*

Example: "When I had to make the presentation to the management team, and my symptoms were so bad I started to perspire, I know that I made myself look like a totally incompetent idiot. What a disaster! All my hard work means nothing!"

7. *Emotional reasoning:* You assume that your negative emotions necessarily reflect the way things really are: "I feel it, therefore it must be true."

   Example: "I would really love to go to that new Italian restaurant that everyone is talking about. But I'm sure I'd have problems if I tried to go, so what's the point?"

8. *"Should" statements:* You try to motivate yourself with "shoulds" and "shouldn'ts," as if you had to be whipped and punished before you could be expected to do anything. "Must" and "ought" are also offenders. When you don't live up to your standards, you feel guilty. When others don't do what they "should" do, you feel anger, frustration, and resentment.

   Example: "I don't know why I can't get through my tax forms without it being such a big production. I should be able to stay organized enough during the year that I don't always end up doing it at the last minute. After all, I am supposed to be an adult!"

   Example: "George should be able to be on time for the movies for once in his life without having to hurry in when the house lights are already down. After all, I manage to be on time and I live further away."

9. *Labeling and mislabeling:* This is an extreme form of overgeneralization. Instead of describing your error in behavioral terms, you attach a negative label to yourself ("failure, screw-up"). When someone else's behavior rubs you the wrong way, you attach a negative label to him/her ("loser, wimp"). Mislabeling involves describing an event with language that is highly colored and emotionally loaded.

   Example: "I had trouble saying what I really felt about the plans to my sister. Just like always, I'm the human doormat."

10. *Personalization:* You see yourself as the cause of some negative external event for which, in fact, you were not primarily responsible.

    Example: "If only I could be more at ease in social events, people would have had a better time at the party. Why am I such a lousy host?"

---

lating helpful responses to problem thinking patterns. As we described in Chapter 2, CALM is a mnemonic for key questions to ask of a negative thought:

C Consequences: Is this thought helping me cope or not?
A Alternatives: What are other ways to interpret the event?

L Logical evidence: How can I collect evidence for or
     against this thought and its alternative interpretation?
M Meaning: What does this negative thought mean to me?

Another way to challenge negative thoughts is to identify and
then target the specific unhelpful cognition. Dispute handles
(Heimberg & Becker, 1984) can be used to challenge negative
thoughts in this way. Examples of IBS-related dispute handles for
specific problem thinking patterns are given in Table 6.3.

Examples from Thought Records completed as self-help assignments are usually helpful in demonstrating the process of
constructing helpful responses. For each automatic thought, a
separate helpful response should be constructed, since individual
Automatic Thoughts have specific content.

Self-help assignments for the week following this and future
sessions should include continued keeping of Thought Records
and Functional Bowel Disorders Diary Forms for IBS Symptoms.
As of this session, columns 4 through 7 of the Thought Record
can now be introduced and assigned. These columns correspond
to steps in the CALM method and the testing of automatic
thoughts. Another possible assignment might also be the cre-
ation of helpful responses for specific hot thoughts identified on
the Thought Record.

Session Theme: Pain Management

Points to cover
- Introduce gate theory of pain.
- Present three distraction methods for pain management.
- Establish a pain baseline; teach Subjective Units of Distress
  Scale (SUDS) self-rating system.
- Relaxation training for pain control.
- Guided imagery for pain control.

Many people with IBS experience high levels of pain, and
this section addresses both the short- and long-term consequences. First, we introduce techniques for coping by teaching
skills that might make it easier for clients to cope with feelings of

TABLE 6.3. Dispute Handles for Specific Problem Thinking Patterns

1. (Apply to *jumping to conclusions*) Do I know for certain that ____ will happen?

    Example: "Do I know for certain that if I go to the dinner, my stomach will rumble so loudly that everybody will hear?"

2. (Apply to *jumping to conclusions* or *all-or-nothing thinking*) Am I 100% certain of these awful consequences?

    Example: "Am I 100% certain that if I decide to tell my friend that she was rude to keep me waiting, she will be so angry that she will never speak to me again?"

3. (Apply to *emotional reasoning* or *disqualifying the positive*) What evidence do I have that ____?

    Example: "Although I usually tend to assume that George will be angry with me if I don't drive him to the cottage, the evidence I have is that Harold used to get angry if I didn't volunteer to drive. What evidence do I have that George will be angry?"

4. (Apply to *all-or-nothing thinking* or *mental filter*) Does ____ have to equal or result in ____?

    Example: "My doctor said that she is pleased with my overall improvement, but she's concerned that I might not be responding well to the new drug she's trying. I guess I'll never find the right treatment!!!"

5. (Apply to *jumping to conclusions*) Do I have a crystal ball?

    Example: "Although I am positive that nobody would want to get involved in a relationship with someone with IBS, can I predict the reaction of every single person I meet over the next 3 years?"

6. (Apply to *catastrophizing* or *all-or-nothing thinking*) What is the worst that can happen? How bad is that?

    Example: "Even if I have to wait 6 weeks to get my tax check back and have to borrow money from my brother, the worst thing that can happen is that he will complain and say I'm irresponsible. How bad has his grumpiness been in the past? Will his remarks totally destroy me?"

7. (Apply to *mislabeling, overgeneralization,* or *personalization*) Could there be any other explanation?

    Example: "Joe looked right through me when I saw him at the conference. Is it because he's decided that I'm a loser, or could it be that he's too vain to wear his glasses in public?"

8. (Apply to *overgeneralization*) What is the likelihood that ____?

    Example: "What is the likelihood that every single time that I go out to lunch I will have to run from the table at least four times and that everybody will notice?"

9. (Apply to *all-or-nothing thinking* or *"should" statements*) Is ____ really so important or consequential?

(continued)

TABLE 6.3. *(cont.)*

Example: "Maybe my feeling that if I don't visit Uncle Bob every day that he is in the hospital and stay for at least an hour, then I am rotten person doesn't make sense, especially if he's sleeping most of the time that I'm there."

10. (Apply to *overgeneralization*) Does _____ 's opinion reflect that of everybody else?

Example: "Just because my coworker Alice thinks that I take too much time planning projects when I could be getting them done doesn't mean that my boss agrees with her; I make a lot fewer mistakes than Alice in the long run."

11. (Apply to *all-or-nothing thinking* or *catastrophizing*) Is _____ so important that my whole future depends on the outcome?

Example: "If that wonderful person I met at the baseball game just wants to be friends, does that mean I'll never find anybody who thinks I'm attractive ever again?"

---

pain and discomfort. Material in this section has been adapted from the work of Keefe, Beaupré, and Gil (1996). We also address longer-term negative consequences of the pain and discomfort of IBS. Clients can make various changes in their lives in an effort to cope. Some of these changes are helpful; others are not. Changes or adjustments can be made in daily activities, such as overall activity level, or doing or not doing specific tasks, bodily responses such as sleep disruption, and changes in thoughts or feelings such as depression, anger, or guilt. Often, responses made to adapt to pain, such as decreasing activity levels, can have long-term consequences such as deconditioning and decreased tolerance for activity. The issue of pain is introduced by first explaining the gate theory of pain.

Possible Script Introducing the Gate Theory of Pain

The gate theory of pain (Melzack & Wall, 1965) states that pain messages originate at the site of bodily damage, injury, or disease and are then passed through a mechanism that works like a "gate to the brain." The brain then interprets the pain message, and it is at this point that pain is experienced. The pain "gate" can be partly or fully opened or closed, determining the amount of pain experienced.

Factors that can open the gate (make pain more central or more intense) include, for example, thoughts that focus attention on the pain, and boredom, because of minimal involvement in life activities. Feelings that can open the gate include depression, anxiety, anger. Behaviors can also open the gate, such as an inappropriate activity level or lack of pleasant activities.

Factors that can close the gate (make pain less central or less intense) include coping strategies such as controlling pain thoughts through attention diversion. Examples of attention diversion are distraction, imagery, and relaxation. Cognitive restructuring strategies, such as altering the self-talk to messages such as "I can handle this, I've handled it before" versus "I can't stand another second of this pain" are also useful. Pain can also be affected by changing activity patterns.

Clients can alter their activity–rest cycling patterns of behavior, as well as instituting pleasant activity scheduling. Descriptions of some of these strategies follow.

Establishing a Pain Baseline Level

At the beginning of sessions focusing on pain, it is helpful for clients to set a baseline pain level by either performing a painful activity for a short period (30 seconds) or by concentrating on painful gastrointestinal symptoms for the same amount of time. Individuals with bowel pain may clench or tense their stomach or belly muscles to initiate or replicate the pain. Immediately thereafter, the therapist can ask clients to rate their highest level of pain experienced. Clients can use a version of the SUDS by rating the pain from 1 (no pain) to 100 (the most intense pain possible). A similar scale will be used for rating anxiety in a later session.

Three Distraction Methods for Pain Management

The therapist can then introduce three distraction methods: focusing on physical surroundings, counting slowly backwards, and focusing on auditory stimuli.

FOCUSING ON PHYSICAL SURROUNDINGS

Clients are instructed that in order to occupy their attention, they should attend carefully to their physical surroundings. They may choose to focus on events, tasks, or objects around them. It is helpful to note that the use of a focal point in Lamaze childbirth preparation helps women cope with labor pain. This example is helpful in normalizing and validating clients' pain. Other examples of focal points may include counting ceiling or floor tiles, examining construction of a piece of furniture, concentrating on a difficult piece of needlework, or a card game. The therapist may wish to bring in a flower or a piece of fruit to serve as a focal point for this exercise.

As a demonstration, ask the client to select some aspect of the physical surroundings in the room and focus on it for 2 minutes. Following this demonstration, ask the client for his/her reactions, and examples when he/she may have used a similar method in day-to-day life.

COUNTING BACKWARDS SLOWLY

Counting backwards slowly is an attention-demanding task. It prevents the attention being focused on pain, which may also promote relaxation. The therapist should ask clients to close their eyes and count backwards slowly from 100 by ones for 2 minutes.

FOCUSING ON AUDITORY STIMULI

Classical music, with its soothing qualities, may be particularly helpful in distracting clients from their pain. To demonstrate the technique, ask clients to close their eyes and listen to three different 1-minute segments of music on cassette tape. Discuss the extent to which clients found some relief from pain through music.

Following these demonstrations, clients select one of these distraction methods and practice it for 30 seconds while doing the same painful activity as earlier. Then, clients are asked to rate the highest degree of pain experienced during the practice of the technique.

The therapist should emphasize the usefulness and importance of practicing these techniques at home and give some assignments using these techniques for clients to perform as behavioral experiments.

Relaxation Training

Relaxation training is widely recognized as being helpful in pain control. Relaxation can break the link between stress and pain, because it counters the autonomic arousal and emotional reactions that have been shown to increase pain. Relaxation also reduces muscle spasm and tension that may increase perceptions of pain. For clients who engage in pain-avoidant abnormal posturing in walking or sitting, relaxation can decrease muscle tension and aid in more normal patterns of movement.

It is important that clients know that they are in control of the timing and level of relaxation during the session. Some clients may wish to keep their eyes open during the practice sessions.

Standard progressive muscle relaxation techniques may be illustrated by the therapist, and clients can then be led through a brief, 20-minute session. Tapes can be provided to clients to facilitate home practice.

Guided Imagery

Along with progressive muscle relaxation, guided imagery techniques may be taught that employ tapes of structured imagery, or the therapist may ask the client to select a scene with personal meaning that is relaxed, safe, warm, and peaceful, and ask the client to "visit" that place for a brief period of time. Having the client attend to a sequence of sensations in the imagined place is helpful. Specifically, the therapist can ask clients to first establish the scene, then ask them to focus on the visual, olfactory, auditory, and sensory (kinesthetic) aspects of the scene by asking a series of questions every 30 seconds or so. The rating of perceived pain before and after this technique may be useful in demonstrating its effectiveness to clients.

Session Theme: Bowel Performance Anxiety

Points to cover

- Explain "vicious circle" model of anxiety.
- Identify trigger situations and/or situations to be avoided.
- Elicit automatic thoughts about trigger situations.
- Create a hierarchy of anxiety-provoking situations.
- Teach techniques for managing anxiety: selective focus, cognitive inoculation.

Individuals with IBS are often hypervigilant to notions of what constitutes socially acceptable behaviors with regard to elimination and digestion. Their beliefs are often perfectionistic, and they may see personal deviation from their standards as shameful. Bowel function is often infused with anxiety. After working with clients with IBS, we have found that a subset have what we term "bowel performance anxiety." The definition that we use for bowel performance anxiety is persistent, distressing apprehension about bowel symptoms in a public context, leading to avoidance of such situations or a heightened state of physiological arousal both before and during such public events.

Treatment Goals

The general goals in working with clients with IBS who suffer from bowel performance anxiety are to decrease the avoidance that many clients experience and also to help them to cope better with their anxiety and the sense of shame they have about such symptoms.

Introducing the "Vicious Circle" Model

We use the following "vicious circle" model with clients to account for bowel performance anxiety. It is important to state explicitly the model of bowel performance anxiety and elaborate on the vicious circle described below. Group members can then consider if this model fits their own experiences.

Clients with IBS have a particular tendency to develop bowel symptoms in response to stress. Other individuals have tendencies to experience stress through other body systems. Clients who are anxious about their bowel performance for an event or in a specific situation, such as during an airplane or car ride, are likely to experience some bowel symptoms in response to their anxiety about bowel function. Because of many clients' perfectionistic beliefs with regard to their bowel function and concern about social desirability, they are likely to devote considerable attention to these symptoms and to make negative predictions with regard to the occurrence of the symptoms. Once the individual focuses on the bowel symptoms and makes catastrophic interpretations with regard to their occurrence, he/she experiences higher levels of anxiety and increased bowel symptoms, forming a vicious circle. In other words, independent of the possible etiological factors in IBS (e.g., enhanced motility and visceral sensation), cognitions such as those mentioned earlier serve to heighten bowel symptoms.

Avoidance of public events and social situations by clients with IBS is common and can produce a significant level of social and occupational dysfunction. It is not uncommon to hear clients' distressing accounts regarding their fears of the annual office picnic or of being invited to dinner at a friend's house. Typically, the anxiety focuses on fears that their bowel will "betray them," and they will be humiliated, miserable, and shamed.

Some clients specifically avoid situations in which their IBS symptoms might be exposed. It is not unusual for clients who avoid or fear exposure in social situations with respect to their IBS symptoms to have had a previous experience in which they felt trapped and exposed in a social situation when they were having IBS symptoms. Frequently, they think of this reference situation when contemplating an excursion or event to which they have been invited.

Some clients, despite their anxiety, force themselves to participate in social events but report high levels of anxiety and lack of enjoyment because of the extensive preparations they have to make before the event and the restrictions that they have to impose on themselves during the event to ensure proper bowel function. In addition, some clients report an increase in bowel symptoms during social occasions.

N. O., a 37-year-old office worker, is quite typical of some clients with irritable bowel symptoms.

Whenever N. O. knew that she would have to attend office dinners, she would try to think of a host of excuses so that she would not have to attend. For two days before the event, she would eat as little as possible in the hope that her bowels would not act up. She would arrive early at the restaurant to find out where the rest rooms were so that she could sit as close as possible to them and sneak out unobstrusively. During the meal, she would pick at the food but would eat very little. If her stomach rumbled, she would feel embarrassed.

Many clients such as N. O. make extensive preparations so that they will not have bowel symptoms. It is not uncommon for them to restrict their food intake in the belief that, if they have not eaten any significant amounts of food, they will not have any noisy or painful bowel activity during the event. Clients with IBS have anxiety about travel on airplanes and buses, or in cars, especially with strangers. Many clients also report anxiety about attending meetings and social encounters. The following are fears that have been elicited from clients with IBS:

Many clients fear experiencing pain or other symptoms that will impair their functioning in a specific situation, so that they will have to reveal their illness. Others fear that they will have embarrassing symptoms, such as noisy bowel sounds or passing gas, which will be noticed by others. Many report concerns that when they use the toilet, they will have such foul-smelling bowel movements that they will embarrass themselves. Some clients fear that their frequency of toilet use will draw attention to themselves. When thinking of social encounters, some clients with IBS fear that they will be trapped in a social situation and have to disclose their symptoms and be humiliated or suffer intense discomfort in silence. Often, clients are afraid that they will not be able to deal with various tasks and challenges because of disabling bowel symptoms.

They fear that those who know of their symptoms will be judgmental and see them as weak and defective, and be rejecting of them.

They believe that they "should" have better control over their bowels and that this lack of control is indicative of personal inadequacy and lack of psychological health. Often, the outside world is seen as harsh, judgmental, and critical.

Identifying Trigger Situations

A useful next step for work with bowel performance anxiety is to ask the group whether there are social situations they avoid or dread because of their irritable bowel symptoms. There are several ways in which a group discussion of this question can help. First, it is helpful for clients to hear that they are not alone in having concerns about negative evaluation because of their symptoms. It is also helpful to know that the same physical symptoms can lead to different degrees of social withdrawal or perhaps no withdrawal at all. A discussion of the common concern of stigmatization because of the symptoms helps to validate their concerns. It is also an opportunity to structure an *in vivo* situation in which clients are able to talk about any embarrassing symptoms in a social situation. Finally, it helps identify for each group member specific triggers that can then be used to elicit automatic thoughts.

Eliciting Automatic Thoughts about the Situations

Eliciting automatic thoughts is important in setting the stage for cognitive restructuring and better coping. A useful exercise for eliciting automatic thoughts regarding bowel performance anxiety and social anxiety is to probe for some of the thoughts that clients had in coming to the initial individual session with regard to how the therapist might react to their symptoms and how they might be evaluated. Similarly, asking clients what preparations they made to ensure their bowels would "cooperate" for the session can begin an exploration of preparations and limitations that are overly restrictive.

It is helpful to ask each group member to recall a specific situation. This helps in the elaboration of the automatic thoughts specific to the individual. As with posttraumatic stress symptoms, recounting the traumatic event in a safe, nonthreatening context can be therapeutic in terms of decreasing the threat of the referent situation.

Cognitive Inoculation

Cognitive inoculation is a set of techniques used to construct cognitive counters to the perceived threat in a situation *before* the actual situation is encountered. Sometimes individuals have little awareness of specific sources of threat in situations, and only know that they are uneasy and anxious. Successful strategies to dispute the validity of the threat are based on a good understanding of the dimensions of the perceived threat. The techniques are the same as those used to dispute automatic thoughts.

This process is called cognitive inoculation because of the parallels with vaccination for illness. It is similar to preparing antibodies against a disease before facing exposure. The individual has the opportunity to prepare disputes to troubling automatic thoughts some time prior to a situation, when anxiety levels or symptoms are minimal. This technique is most effective when individuals actually write down the entire process; it is often quite difficult for clients to remember their helpful responses when they become anxious. Some people find it quite helpful to refer to their written responses for reinforcement during the event itself.

A useful extension of the cognitive inoculation technique is to ask participants to rate their distressing automatic thoughts about potential sources of threat as either *probable* or *possible*. Although there is a wide, if not infinite, range of *possible* catastrophes that might occur in a given situation, most people recognize that the range of *probable* outcomes is much more limited.

Instruct clients to disregard all but the probable outcomes in constructing helpful responses. This helps individuals to recognize the reasonable "limits of worry."

Cognitive inoculation is most effective when used in conjunction with graduated behavioral exposure to situations in which there is the expectation that IBS symptoms will be a problem. The anxiety hierarchy is best employed here to enable individuals to encounter progressively more challenging situations and gain confidence by gathering personally relevant evidence that they can cope with difficult situations.

A next step is to explore the nature of the limitations on the person's life imposed by avoidance and to establish personal goals. This reminds group members of what they have to gain and provides motivation for the anxiety hierarchy.

Preparing Clients for an Anxiety Hierarchy

The third step is to list the situations that are avoided because of IBS-related performance anxieties and to contract with clients ways to decrease the avoidance in a graduated fashion. An anxiety hierarchy is prepared with clients as a structure for doing this. It is a program of graduated exposure to the anxiety-provoking situations. Group members need to be prepared and given tools for coping before they act on the situation in the hierarchy. Cognitive inoculation and distraction are also useful coping techniques for dealing with symptom-provoked anxiety.

Discussing Symptom-Provoked Anxiety

Many individuals with IBS are exquisitely sensitive to internal cues from the gastrointestinal system. Persons who have experienced embarrassment because of IBS in social situations enter such situations highly attuned to any signs that might signal pain or dysfunction of the gastrointestinal tract. Once a change is noted, the focus on this is amplified, and the individual begins to recruit the automatic thoughts outlined earlier. A useful intervention strategy is to try to lessen this internal focus. One rationale that can be used is that this internal sensitivity can be useful for the body to help to alert it to disease or injury but that it can also be unhelpful in contexts where serious disease has been ruled out. The following is a useful behavioral intervention to give clients a greater sense of power of this selective focus. Clients are instructed to monitor their symptoms every 2 or 3 minutes when they are experiencing them, rating them on a severity scale of 1 to 10. On another occasion when they are experiencing symptoms clients are instructed to maintain an external, non-symptom-related focus, such as on the decorations in a room or the topics of conversation in the group. After this, in the debriefing session, it is useful to ask how their symptoms were affected by the two different focus strategies. Many clients report that with the external focus there is a reduction in the degree to which symptoms are obtrusive and disabling. If clients experience symptoms during the therapy session, the therapist may use the opportunity to explore with the client *in vivo* this powerful behavioral intervention of selective focus.

Many clients have not viewed the acknowledgment of symptoms in a social context as acceptable or, if so, only in terms of humiliation. They also have no models of symptom disclosure that are not self-effacing. It is important to explore the belief that having bowel symptoms is shameful. One useful probe is to ask why it is different to have bowel symptoms as compared to discomfort associated with other illnesses such as asthma or arthritis, or other gastrointestinal diseases, such as ulcerative colitis. It is helpful to engage in a role play in which symptoms are acknowledged in a non-self-effacing manner. Working with clients with bowel performance anxiety symptoms can be quite gratifying because of the progress that some individuals make. When clients do not progress, it is important for the therapist to see if they are doing self-help assignments or if he/she has perhaps contracted with them in a too ambitious fashion. Any reservation expressed by clients regarding concerns about experiencing anxiety during exposure can be dealt with by therapists discussing the difference between "productive" versus "unproductive" anxiety. The latter refers to anxiety that is terminated by avoiding and escaping a difficult situation. The former is possible during exposure and refers to the fact that it can be productive to learn and test beliefs about anxiety, which can be used to enable the client to overcome anxiety in the long run (Heimberg & Becker, 1984).

Individuals who are avoiders have spent a great deal of time focusing on scenarios of humiliation, but very little time thinking of how they might cope with symptoms in the fear situation. Clients also often have selective recall for situations where they have not coped well and have felt humiliated. They often poorly recall times they have coped well or when others have been sympathetic about symptoms and nonjudgmental of them. Clients are first helped to recall situations where they have coped well. Clients are taught a variety of techniques to better cope with fear situations. For example, individuals are instructed to utilize their relaxation skills before exposure to decrease the baseline level of anxiety before entering the feared situation.

How to Create an Anxiety Hierarchy

The goal of an anxiety hierarchy is to have clients describe the situations they find most stressful, that is, where symptoms are anticipated to be most problematic. These situations should be ranked in order, from most anxious to least anxious. If participants have difficulty in identifying anxiety-producing situations, they should list those situations that they typically avoid. These may include situations that occur very infrequently (e.g., attending weddings), either because of anxiety about the emergence of symptoms or because they are rare events, but the list should also include more frequently occurring situations (or those that might potentially occur frequently, such as subway travel).

Situations should be concrete ("riding the subway") versus abstract and imaginary ("thinking about my problems"). Participants should be encouraged to specify situations in considerable detail ("riding the subway during morning rush hour, when there are lots of people around"). Clients should use a scale of 1–100 to rate the degree of anxiety or concern about symptoms for each situation. The Subjective Units of Distress Scale (SUDS; see Table 6.4) is useful, with anxiety defined in terms of percent of attention. Note that for this exercise, clients are *not* rating the intensity or pain of specific physical symptoms (gas, cramps); the focus of this scale is on the amount of attention and anxiety focused on the symptoms.

With the completed hierarchy, the therapist can recommend specific behavioral assignments, and the client can see that he/she can make observable progress.

It is possible that there is a "hardwired" response to aversive

TABLE 6.4. Subjective Units of Distress Scale for Anxiety

0–15%: Baseline anxiety

15–30%: Minor attention to symptoms, no disruption of functioning

31–50%: Moderate awareness of symptoms, with normal functioning

51–65%: More than half of attention paid to symptoms, moderate disruption of functioning

66–75%: Considerable distress, normal function only with considerable effort

76–80%: Overwhelming desire to escape

81–90%: Major anxiety, need to escape, minimal functional ability

91–100%: Extreme distress, panic, inability to function

events that may have evolutionary significance: The phenomenon of "one-trial learning" is used to describe animals' reactions to eating poisoned food. Only one such experience is needed for the animal to avoid any such food in the future. Perhaps the experience of gastrointestinal symptoms plays a similar role for some individuals with IBS. Whether or not this is the case, individuals with IBS seem to have little difficulty imagining distressing and embarrassing symptoms occurring in situations in which they have experienced symptoms in the past. In addition, there may be generalization of such concerns to a wide range of similar situations, with every new situation evaluated in terms of its potential for evoking symptoms.

In working with individuals who are not avoidant but nevertheless have high levels of anticipatory and performance anxiety, the goals are to reduce some of the restrictions that they place on themselves. It is important to first explore individuals' specific concerns by collecting automatic thoughts before and during feared situations.

For the first time in 6 months, P. Q. began to eat small amounts of food at a restaurant. "My first thought was that I am going to have to run to the bathroom every 5 minutes and I began to become anxious, but I was able to catch myself and say that I usually eat this much with my family at home without any problem. I still felt a little rumbling in my stomach but it settled and I continued to have my meal."

Anticipatory Anxiety

Just as there are no limits on the imagination, there are similarly no limits on the anticipation of distressing, catastrophic, and humiliating consequences of experiencing IBS symptoms. Clients often provide elaborately detailed descriptions of the anticipated consequences of having symptoms, including the expectation that others observing these symptoms will be contemptuous and judgmental. When individuals begin to ruminate about these anticipated humiliations, they begin to feel physical symptoms of stress. If fact, they might experience higher levels of activation, and concomitant IBS symptoms, *prior* to a stressful event than during the event itself. Anticipatory anxiety is a primary, not a secondary, issue for a substantial proportion of individuals with IBS, who are concerned that their heightened arousal levels will make it more difficult to handle themselves well by increasing the likelihood of IBS symptoms occurring.

> Q. R. experienced a very distressing occurrence a couple of years previously while eating at an unfamiliar hotel restaurant. She almost lost control of her bowels and was unable to find a bathroom. Q. R., a fastidious person, was horrified by the experience and has since been very reluctant to go to unfamiliar places. She listed the following situations as progressively more anxiety producing because of her concern about having to suddenly find a bathroom:
>
> - Eating alone at her desk at work.
> - Eating alone at the local food court where bathrooms were close and available.
> - Eating at the local food court with a friend who was sympathetic to her bowel problems.
> - Eating at a strange restaurant with a sympathetic friend.
> - Eating at a strange restaurant with coworkers who were unaware of her bowel problems.
> - Eating at a strange restaurant with new acquaintances.

In the process of constructing this anxiety hierarchy, Q. R. also was able to access the automatic thoughts associated with each of these situations, some of which were unique to the setting. For example, while eating at the local food court with a friendly coworker, an additional source of anxiety was that her friend would become aware of how stressful the situation was for her and might think she was too emotionally fragile to do her job. Identification of these thoughts was necessary in order to construct effective helpful responses.

In treating Q. R., we encouraged her to systematically encounter these situations, from the least to the most anxiety-producing, in order to gain some evidence about whether her experiences were consistent with her (catastrophic) expectations. The twofold objectives were to gain some firsthand experience that her expectations were, in fact, more negative than her actual experience and to demonstrate that she could manage to endure some anxiety and concurrent sensations of bowel urgency without having an "accident."

During each situation she encountered, she was encouraged to write thought records before and after the event, so she could see whether her negative expectations were met. As she listed anxious expectations prior to the situation, she also worked to counter each anxiety by developing a more helpful response. For example, for the worry that her friend would think it was "weird" to have to get up and go to the bathroom two or three times during the meal, she developed the response that her friend had given many indications that she respected and liked her, and that those feelings would not totally disappear because of her need to go the bathroom frequently. She also practiced some breathing exercises as a way to calm herself and delay her need to use the bathroom. She would often find that if she gave herself enough time to get used to a situation, her sense of bowel urgency would dissipate.

As she practiced encountering the situation that she had previously avoided, she became more confident and more willing to go beyond familiar and "safe" settings. She began to take pride in her accomplishments, and after some weeks of practice, reported that she was able to accept an invitation from her coworkers to go out after work to a bar that she had never gone to before.

A simple example of the relative power of anticipated versus actual anxiety can be seen in the common experience of banging one's shins when getting out of bed to go the bathroom at night.

When this happens, the pain can be intense, and there might be a black-and-blue bruise the next day. It is not so uncommon to forget about the accident, however, and only vaguely recall the circumstances the next day. However, if one were to be told in advance that at precisely 3: 00 A.M. that night he/she would be hit forcefully on the leg with a hammer, it is likely that most of that evening would be spent in wincing anticipation and the notion of being unable to recall the event the next day would be unlikely. It is also likely that the anxiety, worry, and fear would increase the actual pain of the blow.

Anticipatory anxiety is associated with avoidance and/or escape. Both avoidance and escape are powerful learning mechanisms that send the message that the individual is incapable of handling a particular situation (or others like it). The next time a similar situation arises, anxiety levels tend to be higher.

Anticipatory anxiety is also associated with increased sensitivity to small stressors. Things that would ordinarily be taken in stride, such as feeling nauseated, drinking too much coffee, or being in a stuffy room, are piggybacked onto a higher baseline stress level, pushing the person "over the edge," so that IBS symptoms are experienced. Situations that would normally be handled become difficult to get through.

7

Additional Session Themes Related to Coping with IBS

Session Theme: Shame Associated with Having IBS

Points to cover

- Help clients identify social/cultural sources of shame reactions to IBS symptoms, such as the following:

    Nature of IBS as an illness.

    Frustration and behavior of medical doctors.

    Loss of control, which might mean irresponsibility, sloppiness.

    Cultural discomfort with body functions.

- Help clients identify and question the following cognitive sources of shame reactions to IBS:

    Overgeneralization from one problem to a person's whole character.

    Clients' standards of acceptability.

Shame is an important target for intervention for those suffering from IBS. Shame has been defined as a humiliating sense of exposure of central personal inadequacies. Although clients will seldom spontaneously state that they feel shame for having IBS, many aspects of this disorder contribute to a heightened sense of shame. Our clinical experience suggests that shame is an important facet of the hidden suffering of IBS and underlies some of the other IBS-related symptoms of avoidance, depression, and anxiety.

The following are examples of some of the encounters that we have had with clients experiencing strong feelings of shame in our groups.

> R. S., the spouse of a prominent musician, frequently had to entertain guests as R. S. part of her husband's work. She was a meticulous homemaker and always ensured that all aspects of the evening went smoothly. She found such events anxiety provoking and frequently felt that she had embarrassed her husband and failed as a hostess and wife. Her stomach would frequently rumble in what she experienced as a painfully loud fashion. She assumed that guests heard her stomach rumbles but were too polite to ever say anything. She also had to leave the room quite frequently, for whenever she was anxious, she would have mild diarrhea and more frequent bowel movements.
>
> After such parties, R. S. would feel depressed and experience a strong sense of shame. She felt guilty that she could not be a gracious hostess, that her noisy bowel sounds and frequent departures from the living room had made a spectacle of herself and her husband. She was always surprised and somewhat incredulous when guests said how much they had enjoyed the evening.

> T. U., a 33-year-old accountant, found it easier to lie to his friends about the nature of his illness rather than admit that he had IBS. He told them that he had a liver problem. He was certain that his friends would not understand an illness where there was no actual diseased part of his body. He was certain that when he told them that it was a problem for which doctors could not provide a treatment or cure, or find a cause, they would think that it was all in his head. T. U. felt bad about lying but felt that he would be better off hiding what he considered a shameful fact about himself.

U. V. felt it was shameful that she could not control her body better than she did. She related that she had always been instructed in the importance of proper manners and social graces. Until she began to experience IBS symptoms, she had felt proud of her capacity to interact confidently with a great variety of individuals. She was also someone who could balance a busy work schedule and manage the home. She developed IBS during a period of her life when she was under a tremendous amount of pressure trying to balance raising a family and completing a PhD.

Identifying Social Sources of Shame in IBS

Although cognitive-behavioral interventions with issues of shame have not been extensively developed, Klass (1990) describes an approach that is relevant to clinical practice. Some of the interventions that we have used are based on her cognitive-behavioral model for treating shame. Klass stresses the importance of a social learning model of shame. This can be used therapeutically to trace with clients the history of their shame reactions and the types of interpersonal reactions that might have been instrumental in the development of their strong shame response in the first place. "Historical exploration" as a strategy is also discussed in Chapter 2. When clients understand how they learned to appraise IBS in ways that evoke shame, they can begin to question and change those appraisals.

For example, one contribution to shame is the very nature of IBS as an illness. Clients often believe that the lack of a clear physical explanation implies that their symptoms are less real than those of someone who has a more clearly defined disorder such as inflammatory bowel disease. They often feel quite awkward disclosing the nature of their disorder and see this as something akin to admitting they have a personality defect. Often, they are fearful of being judged as defective and have an implicit view of others as disdainful, or at least intolerant of them. Clients often see themselves as defective for having this disorder. Doctors who are frustrated by clients whose symptoms are not easily explained or controlled might inadvertently convey a sense of rejection of the person. Many clients are not given a coherent explanation of IBS as a legitimate disorder, albeit one lacking in tissue pathology or known pathophysiology. Too often, test results that find "nothing wrong" mean that it must all be in the clients' heads and if they had better attitudes or were more disciplined, or were better people, they would not have such symptoms. Lack of an organic cause all too easily gets internalized as a moral deficit or psychological weakness.

One of the most negative aspects of the experience of shame is the sense of isolation that individuals feel. This is compounded by how clients with IBS view issues of control. In general, they view control over many aspects of their lives in particularly positive terms. They view not having control over any aspect of their lives in moral terms and feel a sense of shame with regard to their "loss of control." They also view the world as not being tolerant of imperfect control. Loss of control is synonymous with negative terms such as "irresponsible," "undisciplined," or "sloppy." Many clients find it hard to admit to another person that they have difficulty controlling certain gastrointestinal symptoms. Often, this is experienced by the client as being akin to admitting that they are out of control or not adult. To work with issues of shame, there must be a sufficiently trusting environment so that individuals are willing to risk talking about highly charged areas of perceived personal inadequacy. Individuals often spontaneously talk of the sense of relief they experience in being able to share their feelings of personal shame. The experience of being supported and accepted, despite the "stigma of IBS," helps to diminish the sense that everyone else is critical and rejecting.

Providing clients with a language for talking about "psychosomatic illnesses" and for illnesses without clearly elaborated physical causes is an important step. As mentioned previously, we begin with the presentation of a coherent model of IBS that incorporates both psychosocial and physiological mechanisms. We have found that an important first step for clients is to begin talking about their illness in a non-self-effacing and shaming way.

It is important to acknowledge in the session the ways that certain aspects of bodily functions are not dealt with particularly well in our culture. Our culture and society—through media, popular culture, and everyday discourse—portray as comic or crude the public exhibition of any gastrointestinal functions other than eating. Burping, belching, bowel sounds, and passing gas are all viewed as unacceptable public behaviors to a lesser or greater degree. Individuals who exhibit such behaviors at best are seen as crude and unconventional, and are subject to derision. The therapist might start with a discussion of body odor and the way our society has made sweat and body odor shameful. This can then lead to a discussion of digestive sounds and processes, and the ways our society is not accepting of these bodily processes either.

Questioning Clients' Standards for Acceptable Gastrointestinal Behaviors

It is important to look at the standards that clients have in terms of the range of acceptable gastrointestinal-related behaviors they can permit themselves to exhibit in a public context. Clients suffering from IBS symptoms often feel that they fall outside the acceptable range with regard to their behaviors. The above gastrointestinal-related symptoms represent a shameful departure from acceptable standards of behavior. Even if clients do not in fact have the symptoms described earlier, they often worry about having them or avoid situations for fear that they might occur. Some clients say that it is acceptable to have some symptoms, such as burping, provided that such behavior neither occurs too frequently nor is too loud. Many clients view a rumbling stomach or frequent visits to the washroom as being unacceptable. One question to ask is why certain behaviors are intrinsically more shameful than others.

A suggested area for cognitive-behavioral intervention is to discuss the degree to which failure to meet their standards for acceptable gastrointestinal behaviors warrants the sense of overwhelming shame and denial of self-worth that some clients experience. The purpose of this exercise is to help sensitize clients to their overgeneralization from one behavior to their whole character. Clients who experience shame often have a sense that their area of personal failing outweighs other positive aspects of themselves. One possible intervention is to ask clients to operationalize what makes a person acceptable and worthy. Clients are then asked to rate the degree to which their perceived inadequacy in one area warrants their rejection of other domains of self-worth.

Session Theme: Anger and Assertion

Points to cover

- Introduce signal function of anger.
- Elicit client views about anger expression.
- Identify cognitive triggers for anger.
- Discuss how problem thought patterns can fuel anger.
- Define "assertion" and distinguish from "aggressive behavior" and "nonassertive behavior."
- Help each client develop a hierarchy of difficult situations for acting assertively.
- Role-play examples from clients' hierarchies of difficult situations.

Clients with IBS spontaneously express concerns about how they deal with anger. Nevertheless, this is a potentially fertile area for intervention in terms of clients' IBS symptoms and their general sense of well-being. The relationship of IBS symptoms to clients' difficulties with anger expression is complex. We have observed a number of patterns. For some clients, symptoms occur simultaneously or soon after incidents in which they have suppressed anger. Others are less aware of symptoms at the time but experience them when they engage in ruminative thinking about the incident in which they felt wronged. Still other clients have severe anger outbursts and experience symptoms in the aftermath of these episodes. In many cases, there is no obvious pattern of association of symptoms with anger expression or control.

V. W. illustrates some of these relationships. He experienced a cramping abdominal pain both at the height of his unexpressed anger and afterwards, during periods of rumination. He had come from a family where his father could become explosively angry and often without any provocation. V. W. had always lived in fear of his father's angry outbursts. On several occasions during his teenage years, he had tried to stand up to his father, but the results were extremely negative for him. His father reacted with even greater rage than usual and struck him quite violently on each occasion. Since childhood, V. W. has had a pattern of avoiding conflict and confrontation. On some occasions, as when he had given vent to some of his anger toward his father, he had felt out of control and on the verge of striking out, or throwing and breaking objects. V. W. first began having IBS in the context of a job, where he experienced his supervisor as patronizing, critical, and controlling. He often spent time ruminating about his supervisor, fantasizing the revenge he would wreak on him.

In the therapy sessions, V. W. was able to relate many of the times when there were flare-ups in the symptoms in response to incidents in which he became angry at fellow employees for taking advantage of him or not doing their fair share of work. Typically, he would fume silently in discomfort.

For clients like V. W., there seem to be clear association of symptoms and anger expression difficulties, but for many other clients, the association is not as clear. Before any intervention strategies are introduced, it is important to have a preliminary discussion of the signal function of anger.

Explaining the Signal Function of Anger

Stress to clients that anger itself is not a negative emotion to be suppressed but rather is a useful emotion, providing motivation and forcefulness to our actions if channeled correctly. If not recognized or attended to, anger can lead to problems in interpersonal relationships and possibly physical symptoms in predisposed individuals.

Discussing Views on Anger Expression

After this brief discussion of the signal function of anger, it is important to elicit clients' views about the expression of anger.

Many clients with IBS view anger expression as risky and tend to believe that expressing anger leads to loss of personal control in interpersonal situations. They also worry about rejection and loss of affection and approval if they show any expression of anger, even in the context of firmly expressing a preference or belief.

After finding such connections, some clients are motivated to try to modify how they experience and express anger. Others do not see an association between symptoms and anger expression difficulties. One possible intervention is to ask clients to monitor any changes in the overall level of their symptoms with the use of new ways of dealing with anger expression. Once clients have had a chance to examine any relationship between symptoms and anger expression, the stage is set to begin discussion of alternate strategies for dealing with feelings of anger.

Identifying Cognitive Triggers for Anger

This session then encourages clients to engage in a cognitive-behavioral analysis of anger and irritability problems. Clients are encouraged to recognize the things they say to themselves that may sometimes underlie these reactions. One of the self-exams that therapists may want to try with clients is an irritability quotient. The therapist asks clients to identify how reactive or easily irritated they are by small events. For example, the therapist could describe a situation where someone is picking a friend up at the airport and is forced to wait for a long freight train to pass. The therapist could then ask clients how irritated they would be in this example and begin discussing some of the triggers for angry feelings or behavior. The notion of triggers is very important to this concept, since, in this perspective, thoughts or self-statements are thought to be triggers underlying irritability or angry reactions.

Some Problem Thought Patterns That Fuel Anger

Another important concept is that when people get angry, they blame others. So, for example, people might say, "You are making me angry" or "It's your fault." This session emphasizes the fact that people create their own emotional reactions. In spite of how other people react, it is always up to the individual to determine whether he/she will invoke a type of appraisal that leads to their feeling angry. Once again, the cognitive-behavioral model of events as interpreted by appraisals influencing emotions is invoked. An important point here is that individuals often become angry if they feel that certain things should or should not happen, and that attitudes of this type fuel anger. So, for example, individuals who believe that someone should have done something he/she failed to do, or should not have acted in a certain way, feed reactions that make the target of their behavior angry at them and then blame them. It is important to point out this distinction to clients. Finally, it is important to have clients identify situations in which they have had difficulty with expression of anger. In keeping with the spirit of collaborative empiricism, clients are asked to explore associations between their difficulties with anger expression and their bowel symptoms. As with all the themes discussed in this book, it is important to focus on the person's cognitions as an internalization of cognitions from a larger social context that includes messages about gender role. See Chapter 4 for a discussion of gender role socialization.

As a group, clients with IBS have a great deal of deference to authority and tend to be overly compliant. Often, clients with IBS are concerned with being inoffensive and have a great desire to be liked and accepted. The difficulties they have with anger expression are most often manifested in the form of lack of expression of anger and unassertive behavior. Other clients have difficulty with controlling anger, often after periods of nonexpression of angry feelings.

Teaching Assertiveness Skills

The stage is set for introducing an assertiveness model to clients. In general, the term "assertiveness" is presented as a method of utilizing the signal function of anger to recognize when one feels that one's rights are being infringed upon or threatened.

DEFINING "ASSERTION"

The first step is to introduce the definition of assertion. We use the definition suggested by Lange and Jakubowski (1976) that assertion means standing up for personal rights and expressing thoughts, feelings and beliefs in a direct and honest way which do not violate the rights of others. When successful, both the person who has acted assertively and the individual with whom they have interacted can maintain self-respect. Definitions of aggressive and nonassertive behavior should also be provided to clients.

It is important to solidify the understanding of these three concepts through discussion and rating of specific scenarios. This can be done through discussion of examples provided by Lange and Jakubowski (1976) or through examples elicited from clients. The latter can be more helpful, especially when the materials presented come from their own experience. Clients can then rate the scenarios as assertiveness, nonassertive, or aggressive.

One domain in which most clients have shared difficulties in acting assertively is in getting information and explanations about the diagnosis of their disorder. Many clients find it helpful to discuss these experiences in therapy. The therapist can bring this theme into the therapy session by asking clients to rate their behaviors with respect to assertiveness, nonassertiveness, or aggression, when they interact with medical professionals. It is also helpful to discuss the possible changes clients would like to see in their interactions and to probe for automatic thoughts around what they predict would occur if they changed their behavior in the direction of greater self-assertiveness. For a number of clients, this has emerged as an important target situation in which they have attempted changes in their interactions with their treating physician. For most clients, this is a relatively high-risk situation and such targeting should not be undertaken until after they have attempted less "risky" assertive situations.

HELPING CLIENTS CREATE AND ROLE PLAY A HIERARCHY OF ASSERTION SITUATIONS

To facilitate change and increase the likelihood that clients will attempt new behaviors outside of the therapy session, it is important to develop a hierarchy of assertion situations with increasing risk and difficulty. This is similar to the anxiety hierarchy created for overcoming bowel performance anxiety, described in Chapter 6. The situations in the assertion hierarchy can later be used as graded task assignments (see Chapter 2); in the meantime, role plays of these situations can be an important tool for practicing self-assertion skills. It is important to give clients helpful feedback as to the nonverbal cues associated with their efforts at more assertive behaviors. Modeling of assertive responses is often necessary to help them expand their behavioral repertoires. Many clients with IBS have a good repertoire of skills and are familiar with the concepts of assertive behavior but fail to utilize these skills and concepts because of fears of losing control or retaliation. Over the course of the role plays, clients are asked about their automatic thoughts and alternative responses that increase the likelihood of utilizing their self-assertion skills.

Clients are also asked to attend to emotions and the degree of arousal as they engage in role plays. If they begin to experience high levels of anger and associated cognitions that they are going to lose control, then exercises directed at anger control are necessary. Many clients have difficulty with feelings of anxiety, but instructions to use controlled breathing can reduce the degree of automatic arousal they experience.

> Although T. S. was a very intelligent, thoughtful, and kind person, she felt that she was unable to assert herself in social situations. She believed that she had social "defects" because she was significantly overweight and was reluctant to go to unfamiliar places in case she experienced bowel urgency. Because of these perceived defects, she felt that she had to defer to the convenience and wishes of her friends when making social arrangements. For example, she felt that she usually had to initiate getting together with friends, and that they did not reciprocate equally or would call her at the last minute to make arrangements. She worried that if she asserted her own needs or wishes, that her friends would see her as difficult or demanding and would respond negatively.
>
> In treatment, T. S. became aware of her concern about losing friends, and spent time role-playing expression of her

wishes to her friends in a courteous but firm manner. It was important for T. S. that she not be seen as aggressive or rude, so expressing empathy with the situation of the other person was an important part of the role play. One week, one of T. S.'s school friends visiting from out of town called her on Saturday afternoon and asked to see her that evening. T. S. had to work that night and would have to drive to a distant suburb after she left work to see her friend. She felt a great deal of anxiety when she told her friend that she couldn't see her that evening but was able to tell her friend that she really wanted to spend time with her. Much to her surprise, her friend offered to drive in the next day to see her for brunch. T. S. was pleased that her friend was willing to make an effort to see her; also, she felt relieved at not having to make a long, tiring drive after working her shift. This experience gave her more confidence in telling her friends what arrangements would be convenient for her, and T. S. started to feel less distressed about acknowledging her bowel difficulties to her friends.

As with other cognitive-behavioral interventions, follow-up with self-help assignments is crucial. A common difficulty is that clients take on target scenarios that are too threatening and do not follow through with assignments. Occasionally, clients do encounter some negative consequences over the course of their attempts at assertiveness. Rarely are the consequences as negative as clients had predicted. It is important to elicit these predictions and the results to help put the "setback" in perspective.

It is important to evaluate regularly the changes in clients who engage in more assertive patterns of behavior and how this impacts on their experience of bowel symptoms and general sense of well-being.

Session Theme: Self-Efficacy

Points to cover

- Discuss how predictions about self-efficacy influence actual behavior.

- Identify client beliefs about their self-efficacy.
- Collect data on client beliefs about their self-efficacy.

Research on the effects of self-referent thought in IBS has demonstrated that clients with IBS tend to have lower expectations of their ability to perform behavioral tasks during the presence of symptoms. This predictive relationship seems to hold over time, so that even when symptoms occurred earlier in time, the effects of low performance expectations persist throughout the day. An example here would be an individual who experiences stomach cramps in the morning and decides to excuse him/herself from attending a social event in the evening.

Essentially, the message of this treatment session is that before change can be achieved, a client has to see him/herself as changing. The first step is to examine beliefs about what one can do and what one is limited in doing. The notion of self-efficacy beliefs as targets is an important component in the cognitive-behavioral treatment program, which aims to challenge beliefs regarding somatic cues and their meaning for the client. Assessing positive and negative evidence concerning beliefs about self-efficacy has been useful in treatment. As described by Padesky and Greenberger (1995), this process involves helping the client to muster relevant personal evidence that is first supportive of and then opposed to a particular belief, so that the client can develop a more helpful perspective.

Z. T. started to experience severe stomach pain in a meeting because she had the thought, "I'm not good enough to participate in this kind of meeting." Using a thought record, Z. T. first listed all of the evidence that she could think of that supported her belief that she was not able to participate in meetings, including memories of presenting points of view that were opposed, or experiences when she made presentations that were poorly received. Next, Z. T. listed evidence that did not support the belief that she was not capable, such as receiving positive feedback from others about her arguments and memories of presentations that had been well received. Finally, Z. T. was able to acknowledge that although she was often nervous when presenting her views, in fact, her points were often well received. When she was able to articulate this more balanced view, her anxiety level and her symptoms decreased.

Helping Clients Access Belief-Altering Information

The research on efficacy expectations has shown that these beliefs can be altered through access to four different types of feedback information. The first type is from performance accomplishments, when individuals are able to perform the very behavior they attempt to avoid. The second source of information comes from vicariously observing others perform these behaviors under conditions of stress. Third, verbal persuasion, as exemplified by the psychotherapy situation, has been found useful in changing clients' efficacy expectations regarding specific behaviors. Finally, emotional arousal engendered by a specific event can lead people to push themselves beyond the point at which they feel they will fail. The question of how to incorporate these notions into a treatment session is certainly challenging. The research literature on efficacy expectations can certainly be communicated as part of a rationale for encouraging individuals to test their responses to specific situations. In-session exercises can also be used to show clients how their predictions sometimes serve to limit their behaviors. For example, they can be asked about their initial expectations about therapy and how they feel about therapy at present. Some clients will undoubtedly say that they did not think this treatment would be very helpful to them but now they are finding out interesting things about themselves.

Encouraging clients to self-disclose their expectations can be useful in demonstrating how these beliefs, if adhered to in an absolute fashion, can limit the amount of behavior change they will allow themselves. The client's predictions can be reframed as hypotheses rather than facts. Having clients engage in certain behaviors serves to bring evidence into the session. (See also "Designing Experiments" section of Chapter 2.) The important focus here should be on data-gathering functions rather than verification functions (i.e., whether this is successful or not). The aim is to get clients to consider the possibility that their appraisals are changeable rather than static and fixed. This is an important preliminary step to allowing them to give themselves permission to recalibrate their efficacy expectations.

The following self-efficacy exercise can familiarize clients with their predictions of self-efficacy and the relationship this bears on their performance of behavioral activities. Clients are asked to select a task that they feel would be hard for them to accomplish, as well as a task that would be easy. An example of the former might be something like speaking to a friend about a grievance the client might have felt in the last week, whereas an example of the latter would be buying tickets in advance for a play. The purpose of this exercise is to allow clients to rate themselves on a self-efficacy scale before performing the assignment, then to perform the assignment and rerate their self-efficacy afterwards. The hope is that clients will examine their ratings and notice that after performance of the task, efficacy ratings for the hard task increase such that confidence would be illustrated by higher self-efficacy ratings and they would feel confident doing this task on a future occasion. Ratings for the easy task ought not to change in this way, demonstrating that higher self-efficacy ratings are obtained as a result of successful performance accomplishments. Possible questions or items for the self-efficacy scale would include a confidence scale ranging from 0 (not at all confident) to 100 (extremely confident). Intermediate markers in between would be at 25 (a little confident), 50 (moderately confident), and 75 (quite confident). The first step in constructing an item would be to identify the client's chosen hard and easy tasks. The next step would be to write this task in the following form: How confident are you that you would be able to _____? Or alternatively, if you were thinking of _____, how confident are you that you would be able to do so?

Session Theme: Social Approval and Perfectionism

Points to cover

- Identify and dispute beliefs that self-worth requires social approval.
- Identify and dispute beliefs that only the highest standards (perfection) are "acceptable."

- Distribute and discuss "Helpful Hints for Handling Disapproval."
- Examine and question clients' definitions of "normal" and "abnormal" behavior, and "acceptable" and "unacceptable" behavior.

Many people with IBS believe they must be accepted by others and that they should place demands on themselves in order to be worthy of such acceptance. The heightened need for approval is based upon the assumption that it is necessary for every significant person in one's life to give love, approval, and acceptance in order for one to be happy. This acceptance is conditional upon the individual living up to high standards of behavior in almost every area of life. If these high standards are not attained, the individual will be seen by him/herself (and perceive others as seeing him/her) as unworthy of acceptance. The belief that one *must* be accepted is very different from the acknowledgment that it would be *preferable* to be accepted by other people.

Requiring acceptance as an indicator of one's worth as a person leads to trouble. It causes the individual always to try to please others, often at the expense of his/her own needs. Even if the individual does win the acceptance and approval of significant others, anxiety often accompanies thoughts about the level of effort that is necessary in order to keep this approval. There must be a constant state of vigilance to anticipate the expectations of others. Instead of spending energy deciding what activities are personally fulfilling, enjoyable, educational, or empowering, the individual spends time figuring out other people's expectations.

Some people use the acceptance of others as a way of raising their own self-esteem ("I am only worthwhile if others consider me acceptable"). Gaining *self-respect* involves following one's own interests and learning to like oneself. It also involves a recognition that one has the power to make important personal decisions, and that these decisions are not dictated by the standards of others.

If it is necessary to be competent, well-behaved, and an achiever in order to be accepted by others, the consequences of failure are not just indications of lack of skill or ability in a particular area, but evidence of a basic worthlessness that can lead to rejection by others. Criticism is an indicator that such rejection may be forthcoming. If failure is potentially catastrophic, then criticism is just a precursor of failure and never a source of useful and potentially self-enhancing information. Therefore, the individual is motivated to avoid failure at all costs. This avoidance can lead to a constriction of spontaneous action and risk taking because of fear of making mistakes. Avoidance removes the possibility of being seen as unworthy, but it also makes one's world a smaller, less interesting place.

For individuals with IBS, the significance of all aspects of eating, digesting, and elimination are perceived as linked with self-esteem, so that behaviors that would seem innocuous or mildly embarrassing to many people are devastating to many people with IBS. The belief that "abnormal" eating or bowel habits mean that the individual is also "abnormal" fuels the anxiety that accompanies situations where others can observe IBS-related behavior.

This overemphasis on "normal" versus "abnormal" behavior is very often reflected in a dogmatic rigidity regarding attitudes toward "proper" behavior in virtually all aspects of life. Individuals with IBS are often so immersed in the struggle to live up to rigid standards of conduct that they have little energy left to evaluate whether these standards are personally relevant or fulfilling. The following vignette illustrates the extremely high standards of appearance and behavior that can be observed in some clients with IBS.

> B. A., a 45-year-old woman, held down a demanding secretarial job, while maintaining a well-dressed and carefully groomed appearance. Her weight was right for her height, and she maintained a high level of fitness through exercise. She described herself as a driven workaholic. In the following example, she discusses her concerns about eating in public in a number of settings.

THERAPIST: Let's discuss your anxiety about eating at the lunch meeting at work.

CLIENT: I'm anxious about eating in front of others. I will eat my breakfast at home, and I'll get up very early so I can deal with all my GI symptoms before I get there. I'll just nibble at lunch. I will hardly eat anything.

THERAPIST: What would happen if you ate a lot in a meeting like that?

CLIENT: I don't know because I don't eat a lot with people. When I'm with people I never eat what I would if I'm alone.

THERAPIST: What is the source of stress about going out with someone for a meal and eating a lot?

CLIENT: I always try to have this pretense that I don't eat a lot and that I'm dieting.

THERAPIST: Why.

CLIENT: Because I think I'm fat.

THERAPIST: So when you say eating a lot, what is eating a lot?

CLIENT: What everybody else would consider a normal portion; for me, that is eating a lot.

THERAPIST: Suppose you ate a lot around a friend—what could she think?

CLIENT: Let's go with someone I'm not comfortable with. For example, I was with this woman from work, she's very self-confident and well-put together—the perfect woman. I was intimidated a bit by her. I was feeling really uncomfortable watching her wolf down her meal, and it was just hard for me to eat.

THERAPIST: It was okay for her to wolf it down?

CLIENT: Yes.

THERAPIST: What would happen if you were to wolf it down?

CLIENT: I'm always worried about repercussions from other people. People would think that I eat a lot.

THERAPIST: What would they think?

CLIENT: No wonder she's heavy. I think that's it. I don't have an eating disorder, but I've always strived to work towards this ideal figure that I know I could be if I lost forty pounds.

THERAPIST: (incredulously) Forty!!

CLIENT: Well, maybe ten. I just mind what I eat, especially in public.

THERAPIST: Why especially in public?

CLIENT: Because I'm very much affected by what other people think. The bottom line is that I worry what other people think of me and I've got to learn to say I'm me; this is me; this is what I'm going to eat. Because I often aim to please others and it's stupid because I'm hurting myself.

THERAPIST: That's a good reasonable response.

CLIENT: This is me the way I am. There's always been a drive to be better than everybody. I've got to be better. But again the logical side of my brain says you know you're OK and I just have to learn to listen to that more.

This exchange illustrates the toll that high performance expectations can exert. This young woman preferred to deny herself the right to eat even "normal" amounts of food out of fear of being judged by others. The opinions of others exerted a near-tyrannical power over her, and her drive to push herself to do better than others was essentially a self-protective device. Paradoxically, this drive to achieve more and more (at work, in attaining an ideal figure) tended to increase her arousal level and consequent IBS symptoms, which made her feel more exposed to disapproval. Only by consciously giving herself permission to accept herself relieved her stress level and decreased her symptoms.

Helpful Hints for Handling Disapproval

The following list of "Helpful Hints for Handling Disapproval" contains helpful responses to common negative thoughts. These can help clients dispute these beliefs inside as well as outside the session.

1. Remember that when someone reacts negatively to you, it may be his/her negative thinking that is at the heart of the disapproval.

2. If the criticism is valid, it need not destroy you. You can pinpoint your error and take steps to correct it. You can learn from your mistakes, and you do not have to be ashamed of them. If you are human, then you will make mistakes at times.

3. If you have goofed up, it does not follow that you are a born loser. It is impossible to be wrong all the time, or even most of the time. Think about all the thousands of things that you have done right in your life! Furthermore, you can change and grow.

4. Other people cannot judge your worth as a human being. They can only judge the merit of specific things you do or say.

5. Everyone will judge you differently no matter how well you do or how badly you might behave. Disapproval cannot spread like wildfire, and one rejection cannot lead to a never-ending series of rejections. So even if worse comes to worse and you get rejected by someone, you don't have to end up totally alone.

6. Disapproval and criticism are usually uncomfortable, but the discomfort will pass. Get involved in an activity that you've enjoyed in the past, even though you feel certain it's absolutely pointless to start.

7. Criticism and disapproval can upset you only to the extent that you "buy into" the accusations being brought against you.

8. Disapproval is rarely permanent. It doesn't follow that your relationship with the person who disapproves of you will necessarily end just because you are being criticized. Arguments are a part of living, and in the majority of cases, you can come to an understanding later on.

9. If you are criticizing someone else, it doesn't make that person totally bad. Why give another individual the power and right to judge you? We're all just human beings, not Supreme Court justices. Don't magnify other people until they are larger than life (Heimberg & Becker, 1984).

Perfectionism

In addition to having a high need for social approval, individuals with IBS often struggle with a tendency toward perfectionism in many areas of their lives. Perfectionism is often a characteristic of overdependence on the approval of others. While many people think of perfectionism as being similar to obsessive–compulsive behavior, in fact it more closely relates to the belief that one must be competent and achieve almost everything attempted. In this way of thinking, any failures to achieve the desired standard reflect not only on one's abilities in a particular area, but also on the worthiness of the self as a whole. There is a significant difference between *striving* to be successful and *expecting* that one *must* be successful. Perfectionists live by the adage, "If something is worth doing, it is worth doing well." However, it often takes substantial energy to "do things well" or to feel that a performance meets expectations.

> D. C. borrowed her aunt's cottage for a weekend in order to entertain a group of friends from work. She took the day off work to clean the cottage and to do some cooking for the weekend. Her friends arrived, and things went very well. Everyone had a good time, including D. C. On Sunday afternoon, before they left, everyone pitched in to clean up, and within an hour, the cottage was as clean as when they had arrived. Then everyone but D. C. drove back to the city. D. C., who had been busy making sure that everything went smoothly during the weekend, made herself a drink and collapsed on a deck chair to unwind a bit before heading home. Within 10 minutes, however, she found herself inspecting the cottage and noticing fingerprints on some door handles. Getting out the cleaning supplies, she was soon embarked on "getting things perfect" and was still in a frenzy of cleaning at 10:30 that evening. By the time she got home, she was exhausted, and she started the work week with inadequate sleep and unpleasant bowel symptoms.
>
> When she was asked why she felt it was so important that everything be so perfectly clean, she acknowledged that her aunt probably wouldn't notice all the extra effort she had gone to, especially since she reported that she was happy to have her children play with shells and pebbles on the floor of the cottage living room. She said the cleaning had become obsessive, and she felt obliged to do it to the very best of her ability and to the limits of her strength. She had been raised to show respect by being careful of others'

property, and in her mind, she was thanking her aunt by demonstrating her respectfulness. She equated her meticulous standards of cleanliness with her worthiness as a person. D. C.'s perfectionism and need to put out "110%" was evident in many other areas of her life, and she frequently felt overwhelmed by the many demands she placed on herself. When she felt overwhelmed by responsibilities, her bowel symptoms usually became worse.

In therapy, D. C. was encouraged to purposely set up situations in which she did what she considered to be a less than adequate effort. For example, she gave a dinner party, and rather than have all the food ready before her guests arrived she escorted them to the kitchen and asked them to help set out hors d'oeuvre trays. In discussing this situation in therapy prior to the party, she had anticipated that her guests would be taken aback at her lack of preparedness. In fact, they were relaxed and comfortable, and one guest said that she felt much less nervous at parties when she sat and talked in the kitchen. D. C. was able to see that her guests had a good time even when things were not formal and perfect.

Very often, we see perfectionistic standards applied to bowel performance itself, with individuals having rigid standards of what kinds of bowel behaviors are acceptable or unacceptable.

E. D. became highly anxious whenever she was invited to have dinner at friends' houses. She worried about having to excuse herself two or three times during the course of the evening to use the bathroom and thought that others would think something was wrong. She also worried about causing a foul-smelling odor in the bathroom, or making audible sounds, and feared that others would notice. She agonized about what was a "reasonable" or socially acceptable number of times to use the bathroom during an evening for "normal" people, and was highly conscious of the number of times that others would leave meetings or social events and whether their absence was noted cause for remark. She was not able to disclose her difficulties with IBS to anyone except her husband and sister, even though she had known some of her friends for many years. She believed that if they knew about her bowel problems, they would see her as weak and defective. Her sister was not a very helpful source of support, as she herself was quite sensitive to "unusual" bathroom behavior and would make numerous comments about hearing people make noises in bathrooms.

Over the course of treatment, E. D. was encouraged to participate in social activities, and to use the bathroom as needed. She was also urged to confide her concerns to close friends that she trusted. This was a difficult assignment, since she tended to be quite nondisclosing about any personal issues that she considered to be vulnerabilities. However, she did manage to confide in two close friends, who were supportive of her. She also found that when she did participate in social events, her bathroom behavior did not excite any comments, and some other guests used the bathroom as frequently as she did. On a deeper level, E. D. was able to discuss her low self-esteem and the importance of being accepted by others. She recalled the emphasis that her parents had placed on cleanliness, privacy, and modesty, and the feeling she had gleaned from her parents that bowel functions were fundamentally disgusting and humiliating. Although E. D. continued to struggle with her tendencies toward perfectionism, she became more accepting that her bathroom behavior was within normal limits and even remarked once that "if no one ever made a bad smell in the bathroom, you'd never see an ad for air freshener."

Therapists are referred to Burns (1981) and Antony and Swinson (1998) for a general overview of cognitive-behavioral principles and techniques for overcoming perfectionism. These references include useful discussions on the advantages and disadvantages of being perfectionistic. Several of the behavioral experiments described by these authors serve to change the notion that perfectionism is advantageous. In particular, one self-help assignment that may be especially helpful to clients with IBS is to test their negative conceptions about being average or less than perfect by deliberately seeking to be as average as possible for a given period of time. This exercise serves as a behavioral disconfirmation of clients' negative expectations about being average and can demonstrate some advantages. Clients can be encouraged to generate (in session) more helpful self-evaluative standards. The quest for alternative standards can be promoted by considering the standards clients use in evaluating individuals whom they admire, but who are not perfect (or superior to others). Frequently, we have found that these other-referent criteria involve personal qualities unrelated to rank or outcome.

Session Theme: Control

Points to cover

- Question whether "control" is always positive.
- Question whether "control" is always possible.
- Examine beliefs about loss of control and shame.
- Examine the paradox of control: Too much control can result in loss of control; less control may result in more effective control.

Control is a prominent theme among clients with IBS. Individuals with IBS perceive themselves as being controlled by their symptoms, with their symptoms making it impossible for them to behave spontaneously or without elaborate preparations and safeguards. When symptoms flare up, IBS sufferers often describe the most catastrophic consequences in terms of losing control: losing control of their bowels, being unable to delay using the bathroom, or being unable to mask or ignore their symptoms. This loss of control is very often associated with an inability to hide the "shameful" symptoms from others, and the sense of loss of control is connected with a sense of loss of social competence.

Individuals with IBS often respond to their symptoms by trying to control aspects of the environment that may be associated with symptoms. They often develop quite elaborate systems of environmental control, such as establishing rigid routines of eating or not eating before social events, restricting activities to settings where the locations of bathrooms is known, or traveling to places only along certain well-researched routes. These routines may become extremely ritualized and place severe limitations on the freedom of movement of the IBS sufferer. Individuals with IBS often avoid eating outside their homes, taking car trips, or attending movies or concerts.

Possible Script Introducing Control

The unquestioning assumption that control is a positive characteristic is shared by many people in our society. The image of the person who "has it all under control" tends to be favorable, and we see such a person as calm, self-confident, and capable. Often, the process of becoming an adult is seen as the process of obtaining more and more control over our lives: We control our impulse spending better; we can make more choices as to the kind of work we do; we become more self-disciplined about our personal habits. When we think of someone who is "out of control," we think of a child having a tantrum, an adolescent who can't handle new freedoms, or a drunk partygoer who is behaving badly.

One of the reasons that control is viewed so positively is that being in control is associated with making choices. We're used to observing how things work, or what the rules are, and then acting so as to have more control over our environment and increase our choices. Most of the time, this pays off. For example, if we can control our work schedule, we can avoid commuting in rush-hour traffic. Or if we observe the unwritten rule of addressing the police officer who pulls us over as "officer" instead of "Bozo," the consequences are much more likely to be positive. Usually, the greater the awareness of the rules, the more control we have, and the more positive the consequences.

When we can't control external circumstances, we feel buffeted by events, out of control, and vulnerable.

However, sometimes our expectations of being in control are not helpful. We may feel that we have prepared for every contingency for our vacation—and then a hurricane strikes. Or we may try to anticipate our boss's every response to our request for a raise—only to hear that the business is closing. It's almost impossible to predict the curve balls that life will throw at us, no matter how hard we try to plan for every eventuality. In addition, it may not be helpful or desirable to be in control of all aspects of our life. For example, we can choose to control the rate of our breathing while we are conscious, but would we want to spend so much of our attention managing something that could as easily go on "automatic pilot"? Similarly, although it is possible to have some control over bowel functions, such as being able to delay bowel movements, we usually encounter fewer difficulties when we allow our body to find a routine that works for it. By exerting too much control, such as delaying bowel movements too long, we find that we actually create difficulties for ourselves.

Sometimes the best that we can do is to be reasonably prepared for the most likely events, and to handle the things that come up unexpectedly as best we can at the moment. And usually, our ad hoc responses are good enough. If we have enough confidence in our ability to handle the unexpected, the burden of planning and preparing for every eventuality becomes much lighter.

> F. E., a consultant, is obliged to participate in many business lunches. She worries about having to use the bathroom several times during these lunches and fears that her clients will see this behavior as abnormal. A sample of her automatic thoughts follows:
>
> "Since I am selling my expertise, my clients need to see me as relaxed, confident, and in control."
> "If I have to run to the bathroom frequently, they will see this behavior as abnormal, and see me as being unable to control myself."
> "If I can't control my body, they will think I can't control my emotions, that I get overwhelmed with any responsibilities."
> "The extent to which I am seen as being in control of all aspects of my life is how my competence is judged."
> "If I am seen as not in control of any part of my life, including my bowels, I will be seen as incompetent and worthless."

In addition to the way the issue of control is related specifically to symptoms, control seems to be a prominent feature of the personality styles of many clients with IBS. They often seem to spend a great deal of energy living up to social expectations. Many clients are compliant, conscientious, and well-mannered. They work hard at maintaining standards of behavior in their work and personal lives and are often sensitive to hierarchical differences in power and authority. They value being in control and tend to view others' weakness unsympathetically and their own weakness critically. This focus on control is sometimes striking: One client who was describing her symptoms during an initial interview used the word "control" more than 90 times during a 1-hour interview.

Helping Clients Examine the Paradox of Control

A major task of therapy is to examine the following paradox: Often, the driving need to exert control (over symptoms or the environment) results in the constriction of movement and the loss of freedom of choice—in other words, a loss of control. Indeed, one of the goals of therapy is to restore spontaneity to clients who have labored under such restrictions, so that they are able to go out, to eat when they are hungry, and give themselves permission to be less focused on their symptoms. Major indicators of progress are clients' reports that they can "relax the reins" a little and allow their bodies to establish their own natural cycles. It is perhaps noteworthy that the processes of digestion and elimination are primarily under control of the autonomic nervous system, which is capable of operating when there is no conscious process of control whatsoever.

This process can best be accomplished by examining what aspects of bowel functioning are facilitated by using cognitive-behavioral techniques to establish helpful expectations for control over bowel functions. For example, individuals may have to tell themselves that it is normal for stomachs to rumble when people are hungry or have just eaten; or that it is possible to be a socially valued person if one has to use the restroom two or three times during a meal. The catastrophic nature of automatic thoughts associated with bowel symptoms must be explored and unhelpful thoughts discussed. Such a process occurs most effectively when it is carried out as a systematic element of progressive behavioral exposure. In addition to the symptom hierarchies described earlier, clients can sometimes define challenging situations in terms of control itself; that is, they can differentiate situations on the basis of how much environmental control they feel impelled to exert and make a conscious effort to exert less control. This method can also serve to define stressful situations associated with the onset of symptoms in ways that may be psychologically more coherent than seemingly more explicit behavioral or situational definitions. It also taps into clients' creativity in coming up with individually meaningful ways of relaxing control. One client, for example, noted that she held on to a sense of control by maintaining tense muscle tone in her abdomen. When she made the decision to release control, she found that her breathing techniques became more successful as an intervention.

8

Final Session

Therapy Termination

Termination in a brief therapy is extremely important to ultimate outcome. Beck (1976) discusses termination as key in determining how clients use skills learned in therapy. We agree that termination of the therapy deserves special attention just as socialization to therapy deserved special attention at the beginning of therapy. Termination is not just the end of therapy; it is also the beginning of a different phase of independent experimentation and learning by clients with regard to concepts and skills acquired over the course of therapy.

Termination Begins with the Beginning

One of the key elements in consideration of termination in cognitive-behavioral treatment of IBS is that termination begins with the first session. It is important to reintroduce to clients the fact that this is a short-term therapy and to allow time for exploration of their reactions and beliefs about the short-term nature of the intervention in the first session. Initially, some clients see the fact that therapy will last only 12 sessions in positive terms. To them, the fact that therapy is brief indicates that they will make rapid progress.

Other clients may be somewhat skeptical about the value of the treatment. Not yet invested in the process, they have not yet developed strong feelings and attitudes regarding the duration.

Termination Anxieties

As therapy progresses, clients often become aware of the progress that they are making. There is an associated change in clients' attitudes toward termination. The following are some of the attitudes and beliefs expressed by clients with regard to termination. Often, they will begin to express some regret about the brevity of therapy. Usually there are different anxieties embedded in this concern. Individuals who have made some gains believe that if therapy were longer, they could make greater gains. Others wonder whether gains will be maintained without the support of the therapist and the structure of the sessions. There is concern about separation from the therapist and therapy.

It is important to be aware that these shifts are occurring. In order to tap into this change, it is necessary to probe on multiple occasions over the 12 sessions the client's feelings and beliefs regarding termination. This is best done in the context of periodic reminders of the number of sessions left in the therapy protocol.

> H. G. had made some gains in dealing with avoiding public situations where she might have difficulty finding a bathroom, but she had not made the gains that she envisioned for herself when she composed her hierarchy of anxiety-provoking situations. She felt discouraged as therapy was coming to an end. The following automatic thoughts were elicited: "I didn't get very far through the therapy," "I'll never have a normal life." It was helpful to review with her some of the items that she had crossed off her avoidance hierarchy. She was able to accept that she hadn't achieved as much as she had hoped for in therapy, but nevertheless, she could continue to work through the hierarchy on termination of the sessions. She admitted that her lack of "total success" was hard for her to accept and that she would have to remind herself on a regular basis of some of her achievements to avoid discouragement.

Does the Need for More Help Mean Failure?

Some individuals have the notion that once the cognitive-behavioral therapy has ended, they have to function autonomously without any further assistance or therapy.

For many individuals who have IBS, participating in cognitive-behavioral therapy may be the first time they have framed their problems in psychological terms. Some see cognitive-behavioral therapy as their "chance" to deal with these concerns. For these clients, termination of therapy may mean that they cannot avail themselves of further psychological help. As therapy progresses, individuals may have greater awareness of areas of psychological stress and conflict, which leads to increased anxiety about termination, especially if paired with the belief that they have to cope using only their own resources. It is helpful for such clients to underscore the progress they have made in better identifying areas of stress and learning skills to cope with areas of stress and conflict. It is important to explore client beliefs and attitudes toward further therapy should this prove necessary. We have found that clients' termination anxiety is decreased if they are able to see the possibility of seeking further assistance in the future should they reach such an impasse. It is also important to provide concrete information as to how such help might be obtained if needed.

> In therapy, I. H. became increasingly aware of the dissatisfaction she experienced in relation to her husband. What she had experienced previously as justifiable criticism of her inadequacies, she now experienced as unwarranted and controlling behavior on his part. Over the course of treatment, she began to relate to her husband in a more assertive manner but also found that there was increased tension between them. I. H. began to consider trying to convince her husband to enter marital therapy with her. As part of the termination, I. H. was given the name of several possible marital therapists and also was encouraged to phone if these did not work out. I. H. hoped that the relationship with her husband might change if she consistently related to him in a more assertive fashion. She was also relieved by the suggestions regarding help.

Termination Predictions

As Beck et al. (1979) emphasizes, in cognitive therapy for depression, it is important to elicit automatic thoughts about termination and to treat them as predictions that are subject to testing through looking at alternatives.

> As an example, I. H. predicted that she would never be able to deal with conflict without the help of the therapist. This was elicited early in the course of treatment, after the modules dealing with assertiveness and anger expression. A series of experiments were designed to test out this hypothesis that she couldn't deal with conflict without the therapist. I. H. was able to reframe her original prediction with the statement that although she found the therapist's input helpful, she could manage with most situations on her own.

The Last Session

The last session of therapy ends the termination process and is a time for clients and therapist to wrap up loose ends and say good-bye, but, as outlined earlier, it forms only an element of the termination process. Part of the session may be used to review gains made in therapy and areas in which clients' efforts will be directed for continuing progress.

It is important to leave adequate time for actually saying good-bye and processing some of the feelings that both clients and therapist have about ending therapy. It is important not to underestimate the sadness that some clients have about the end of therapy, where they have had support and a safe environment to talk about potentially painful and shameful topics.

Conclusion

This book has highlighted an empirically tested cognitive-behavioral protocol for clients with IBS from our Toronto group. We have provided information regarding practical assessment and treatment issues with possible scripts and case examples for health professionals to use to identify and highlight factors that may arise in working with clients with IBS relative to other clinical groups. Results from our research protocol indicate that cognitive-behavioral group therapy significantly reduces depressive symptoms, need for social desirability, and gastrointestinal symptoms that include abdominal pain, tenderness, diarrhea, constipation, and bloating. These psychological and gastrointestinal symptoms did not improve in the control groups. While these results, together with previous work, are promising, future work is needed to further refine the model and specific techniques and strategies to increase the efficacy of cognitive-behavioral therapy for IBS.

APPENDIX 1

Functional Bowel Disorders
Diary Form

Week No. _____ Client Initials _____ ID No. _____

INSTRUCTIONS: Please fill out diary every night. Record information from the previous 24 hours.

Question 1. Write the total number of bowel movements in blank.

Question 2. Use the number from the list below that best describes your bowel movements:
1. Separate hard lumps, like nuts
2. Sausage shaped but lumpy
3. Like a sausage or snake, with cracks on its surface
4. Like a sausage or snake, smooth and soft
5. Soft blobs with clear-cut edges
6. Fluffy pieces with ragged edges, mushy
7. Watery, no solid pieces
8. None

Question 3: Circle the number that best describes the amount of pain you felt today.

Day 1: Date _____

1. Number of bowel movements ____
2. Description (use number from above) ____
3. Pain: (1) none (2) mild (3) moderate (4) severe (5) very severe

Day 2: Date _____

1. Number of bowel movements ____
2. Description (use number from above) ____
3. Pain: (1) none (2) mild (3) moderate (4) severe (5) very severe

Day 3: Date _____

1. Number of bowel movements ____
2. Description (use number from above) ____
3. Pain: (1) none (2) mild (3) moderate (4) severe (5) very severe

Day 4: Date _____

1. Number of bowel movements ____
2. Description (use number from above) ____
3. Pain: (1) none (2) mild (3) moderate (4) severe (5) very severe

---

Note. From Drossman (1995a).

Day 5: Date _____

    1. Number of bowel movements ____
    2. Description (use number from above) ____
    3. Pain: (1) none (2) mild (3) moderate (4) severe (5) very severe

Day 6: Date _____

    1. Number of bowel movements ____
    2. Description (use number from above) ____
    3. Pain: (1) none (2) mild (3) moderate (4) severe (5) very severe

Day 7: Date _____

    1. Number of bowel movements ____
    2. Description (use number from above) ____
    3. Pain: (1) none (2) mild (3) moderate (4) severe (5) very severe

Day 8: Date _____

    1. Number of bowel movements ____
    2. Description (use number from above) ____
    3. Pain: (1) none (2) mild (3) moderate (4) severe (5) very severe

Day 9: Date _____

    1. Number of bowel movements ____
    2. Description (use number from above) ____
    3. Pain: (1) none (2) mild (3) moderate (4) severe (5) very severe

Day 10: Date _____

    1. Number of bowel movements ____
    2. Description (use number from above) ____
    3. Pain: (1) none (2) mild (3) moderate (4) severe (5) very severe

APPENDIX 2

Thought Record

1. Situation	2. Moods	3. Automatic Thoughts (Images)	4. Evidence That Supports the Hot Thought	5. Evidence That Does Not Support the Hot Thought	6. Alternative/ Balanced Thoughts	7. Rate Moods Now
Who were you with? What were you doing? When was it? Where were you?	Describe each mood in one word. Rate intensity of mood (0–100%).	What was going through my mind just before I started to feel this way? What does this say about me? What does this mean about me? my life? my future? What am I afraid might happen? What is the worst thing that could happen if this is true? What does this mean about how the other person(s) feel(s)/think(s) about me? What does this mean about the other person(s) or people in general? What images or memories do I have in this situation?	Circle hot thought in previous column for which you are looking for evidence. Write factual evidence to support this conclusion. (Try to avoid mind-reading and interpretation of facts.)	Ask yourself the questions in the Hint Box (p. 70) to help discover evidence which does not support your hot thought.	Ask yourself the questions in the Hint Box (p. 95) to generate alternative or balanced thoughts. Write an alternative or balanced thought. Rate how much you believe in each alternative or balanced thought (0–100%).	Copy the feelings from Column 2. Rerate the intensity of each feeling from 0 to 100% as well as any new records.

Note. From Greenberger and Padesky (1995). Page numbers on the Thought Record refer to page numbers there. Copyright 1995 by The Guilford Press. Reprinted by permission.

References

Abbey, S. E., & Garfinkel, P. E. (1991). Neurasthenia and chronic fatigue syndrome: The role of culture in the making of a diagnosis. *American Journal of Psychiatry, 148,* 1638–1646.

Akman, D., & Toner, B. B. (1999). *Including families in the treatment of irritable bowel syndrome.* Unpublished manuscript.

Ali, A., Richardson, D. C., & Toner, B. B. (1998). Feminine gender role and illness behaviour in irritable bowel syndrome. *Journal of Gender, Culture, and Health, 3,* 59–65.

Ali, A., & Toner, B. B. (1996a). Sexual abuse and self-blame in women with irritable bowel syndrome. *Psychosomatic Medicine, 58,* 66.

Ali, A., & Toner, B. B. (1996b, June 20). *Emotional abuse and self-silencing in women with irritable bowel syndrome.* Paper presented at the 22nd Annual Department of Psychiatry Research Day, University of Toronto.

Ali, A., Toner, B. B., Stuckless, N., Gallop, R., Diamant, N. E., Gould, M. I., & Vidins, E. I. (in press). Emotional abuse, self-blame and self-silencing in women with irritable bowel syndrome. *Psychosomatic Medicine.*

Antony, M. M., & Swinson, R. P. (1998). *When perfect isn't good enough: Strategies for coping with perfectionism.* Oakland, CA: New Harbinger.

Arn, I., Theorell, T., Uvnas-Moberg, K., & Jonsson, C. (1989). Psychodrama group therapy for patients with functional gastrointestinal disorders. *Psychotherapy and Psychosomatics, 51,* 113–119.

Barnett, L. R. (1986). Bulimarexia as symptom of sex role strain in professional women. *Psychotherapy, 23,* 311–315.

Barsky, A. J., Geringer, E., & Wool, C. A. (1988). A cognitive-educational treatment for hypochondriasis. *General Hospital Psychiatry, 10,* 322–327.

169

Beck, A. T. (1976). *Cognitive therapy and the emotional disorders*. New York: International Universities Press.

Beck, A. T., Emery, G., & Greenberg, R. (1985). *Anxiety disorders and phobias: A cognitive perspective*. New York: Basic Books.

Beck, A. T., Rush, A. J., Shaw, B. F., & Emery, G. (1979). *Cognitive therapy of depression*. New York: Guilford Press.

Beitchman, J. H., Zucker, K. J., Hood, J. E., daCosta, G. A., Akman, D., & Cassavia, E. (1992). A review of the long-term effects of child sexual abuse. *Child Abuse and Neglect, 16*, 101–118.

Bennett, P., & Wilkinson, S. (1985). A comparison of psychological and medical treatment of the irritable bowel syndrome. *British Journal of Clinical Psychology, 24*, 215–216.

Bepko, C., & Krestan, J. (1990). *Too good for her own good*. New York: Harper & Row.

Bernstein, D. A., & Borkovec, T. D. (1973). *Progressive relaxation training: A manual for the helping professions*. Champaign, IL: Research Press.

Blanchard, E. B., Greene, B., Scharff, L., Schwarz-McMorris, S. P. (1993). Relaxation training as a treatment for irritable bowel syndrome. *Biofeedback and Self-Regulation, 18*, 125–132.

Blanchard E. B., Scharff L., Schwarz, S. P., Suls, I. N., & Barlow, D. H. (1990). The role of anxiety and depression in the irritable bowel syndrome. *Behavior Research and Therapy, 28*, 401–405.

Blanchard, E. B., Schwarz, S. P., Suls, J. M., Gerardi, M. A., Scharff, L., Greene, B., Taylor, A. E., Berreman, C., & Malamood, H. S. (1992). Two controlled evaluations of a multicomponent psychological treatment of irritable bowel syndrome. *Behaviour Research and Therapy, 2*, 175–189.

Blechman, E. (1984). Women's behavior in a man's world: Sex differences in competence. In E. Blechman (Ed.), *Behavior modification with women*. New York: Guilford Press.

Borkovec, T. D., & Nau, S. D. (1972). Credibility of analogue therapy rationales. *Journal of Behavior Therapy and Experimental Psychiatry, 3*, 257–260.

Brewin, C. R., Andrews, B., & Gotlib, I. H. (1993). Psychopathology and early experience: A reappraisal of retrospective reports. *Psychological Bulletin, 113*, 82–98.

Briere, J., & Runtz, M. (1990). Differential adult symptomatology associated with three types of child abuse histories. *Child Abuse and Neglect, 14*, 357–364.

Broverman, I., Broverman, D., Clarkson, F. E., Rosenkrantz, P., & Vogel, S. (1970). Sex role stereotypes and clinical judgments of mental health. *Journal of Personality and Social Psychology, 34*, 1–7.

Browne, A., & Finkelhor, D. (1990). Initial and long-term effects: A review of the research. In D. Finkelhor (Ed.), *A sourcebook of child sexual abuse*. Beverly Hills, CA: Sage.

Buchanan, D. C. (1978). Group therapy in chronic physically ill patients. *Psychosomatics, 19*, 425–431.

Burns, D. D. (1981). *Feeling good: The new mood therapy.* New York: Signet.

Burns, D. D., & Nolen-Hoeksema, S. (1991). Coping styles, homework assignments and the effectiveness of cognitive behavioral therapy. *Journal of Consulting and Clinical Psychology, 59,* 564–578.

Burns, D. G. (1986). The risk of abdominal surgery in irritable bowel syndrome. *South African Medical Journal, 70,* 91.

Chabbra, M., Toner, B. B., Ali, A., & Stuckless, N. (1999). *The relationship between somatic symptoms and the attribution of illness in irritable bowel syndrome patients.* Unpublished manuscript.

Chesler. P., (1972). *Women and madness.* New York: Doubleday.

Colgan, S., Creed, F. H., & Klass, S. H. (1988). Psychiatric disorder and abnormal illness behavior in patients with upper abdominal pain. *Psychological Medicine, 18,* 887–892.

Corney, R. H., & Stanton, R. (1990). Physical symptom severity, psychological and social dysfunction in a series of outpatients with irritable bowel syndrome. *Journal of Psychosomatic Research, 34,* 483–491.

Corney, R. H., Stanton, R., Newell, R., Clare, A., & Fairclough, P. (1991). Behavioral psychotherapy in the treatment of irritable bowel syndrome. *Journal of Psychosomatic Research, 35,* 461–469.

Cosentino, F., & Heilburn, A. B., Jr. (1964). Anxiety correlates of sex-role identity in college students. *Psychological Reports, 14,* 729–730.

Covi, L., & Lipman, R. (1987). Cognitive behavioral group psychotherapy combined with imipramine in major depression. *Psychopharmacological Bulletin, 23,* 173–176.

Covi, L., & Primakoff, L. (1988). Cognitive group therapy. In A. J. Frances & R. F. Hales (Eds.), *Annual review of psychiatry* (Vol. 7). Washington, DC: American Psychiatric Association Press.

Covi, L., Roth, D., & Lipman, R. S. (1982). Cognitive group psychotherapy of depression: The closed-ended group. *American Journal of Psychotherapy, 36,* 459–469.

Craig, T. K. G., & Brown, G. W. (1984). Goal frustration and life events in the aetiology of painful gastrointestinal disorder. *Journal of Psychosomatic Research, 28,* 411–421.

Creed, F., Craig, T., & Farmer, R. (1988). Functional abdominal pain, psychiatric illness, and life events. *Gut, 29,* 235–242.

Crowne, D., & Marlowe, D. (1960). A new scale of social desirability independent of psychopathology. *Journal of Consulting Psychology, 24,* 349–354.

Davis, D., & Padesky, C. (1989). Enhancing cognitive therapy with women. In A. Freeman, K. Simon, L. Beutler, & H. Arkowitz (Eds.), *Comprehensive handbook of cognitive therapy.* New York: Plenum Press.

Deaux, K. (1984). From individual differences to social categories: Analysis of a decade's research on gender. *American Psychologist, 39,* 105–116.

Domino, J. V., & Haber, J. D. (1987). Prior physical and sexual abuse in women with chronic headache: Clinical correlates. *Headache, 27,* 310–314.

Drossman, D. A. (1995a). *Functional Bowel Disorders Diary Form.* Unpublished manuscript.

Drossman, D. A. (1995b). Psychosocial factors in the care of patients with gastrointestinal disorders. In T. Yamada (Ed.), *Textbook of gastroenterology*. Philadelphia: Lippincott.

Drossman, D. A. (1996). Gastrointestinal illness and the biopsychosocial model [Editorial]. *Journal of Clinical Gastroenterology, 22*, 252–254.

Drossman, D. A. (1998). Presidential address: Gastrointestinal illness and biopsychosocial model. *Psychosomatic Medicine, 60*, 258–267.

Drossman, D. A., Creed, F. H., Fava, G. A., Olden, K. W., Patrick, D. L., Toner, B. B., & Whitehead, W. E. (1995). Psychosocial aspects of the functional gastrointestinal disorders. *Gastroenterology International, 8*, 47–90.

Drossman, D. A., Creed, F. H., Olden, K. W., Svedlund, J., Toner, B. B., & Whitehead, W. E. (1999). Psychosocial aspects of the functional gastrointestinal disorders. *Gut, 45*(Suppl. 2), 1125–1130.

Drossman, D. A., Leserman, J., Nachman, G., Li, Z., Gluck, H., Toomey, T. C., & Mitchell, C. M. (1990). Sexual and physical abuse in women with functional or organic gastrointestinal disorders. *Annals of Internal Medicine, 113*, 828–833.

Drossman, D. A., Li, Z., Andruzzi, E., Temple, R. D., Talley, N. J., Thompson, W. G., Whitehead, W. E., Janssens, J., Funch-Jensen, P., Corazziari, E., Richter, J. E., & Koch, G. G. (1993). U.S. householder survey of functional gastrointestinal disorders: Prevalence: Sociodemography and health impact. *Digestive Disease Science, 38*, 1569–1580.

Drossman, D. A., Li, Z., Leserman, J., Toomey, T. C., & Hu, Y. (1996). Health status by gastrointestinal diagnosis and abuse history. *Gastroenterology, 110*, 999–1007.

Drossman, D. A., McKee, D. C., Sandler, R. S., Mitchell, C. M., Cramer, E. M., Lowman, B. C., & Burger, A. L. (1988). Psychosocial factors in the irritable bowel syndrome: A multivariate study of patients and nonpatients with irritable bowel syndrome. *Gastroenterology, 95*, 701–708.

Drossman, D. A., Richter, J. E., Talley, N. J., Thompson, W. G., Corazziari, E., & Whitehead, W. E. (1994). *Functional gastrointestinal disorders: Diagnosis, pathophysiology and treatment*. Boston: Little, Brown.

Drossman, D. A., Sandler, R. S., McKee, D. C., & Lovitz, A. J. (1982). Bowel patterns among subjects not seeking health care. *Gastroenterology, 83*, 529–534.

Drossman, D. A., Whitehead, W. E., & Camilleri, M. (1997). Medical position statement: Irritable bowel syndrome. *Gastroenterology, 112*, 2118–2119.

Ellis, A., & Dryden, W. (1987). *The practice of rational–emotive therapy*. New York: Springer.

Emmott, S. D. (1994). The CALM method of helpful responses. In B. B. Toner, Z. V. Segal, S. D. Emmott, & D. Myran. *Cognitive-behavioral treatment manual for functional bowel disorders*. Unpublished manual.

Engel, G. L. (1977). The need for a new medical model: A challenge for biomedicine. *Science, 196*, 129–136.

Fabrega, H., Jr. (1991). Somatization in cultural and historical perspective.

In L. Kirmayer & J. M. Robbins (Eds.), *Current conceptions of somatic disorders*. Washington, DC: American Psychological Association Press.

Falloon, I. R. H. (1991). Behavioral family therapy. In A. S. Gurman & D. P. Kniskern (Eds.), *Handbook of family therapy* (Vol. II). New York: Brunner/Mazel.

Feather, N. T., & Simon, J. G. (1975). Reactions to male and female success and failure in sex-linked occupations: Impressions of personality, causal attributions, and perceived likelihood of different consequences. *Journal of Personality and Social Psychology, 31*, 20–31.

Felitti, V. J. (1991). Long-term medical consequences of incest, rape and molestation. *Southern Medical Journal, 84*, 328–331.

Fodor, I. E. (1974). Sex role conflict and symptom formation in women. *Psychotherapy, 11*, 22–29.

Ford, M. J., Miller, P. M., Eastwood, J., & Eastwood, M. A. (1987). Life events, psychiatric illness and the irritable bowel syndrome. *Gut, 28*, 160–165.

Franks V., & Rothblum, E. D. (1983). *The stereotyping of women: Its effects on mental health*. New York: Springer.

Gall, M. D. (1969). The relationship between masculinity–femininity and manifest anxiety. *Journal of Clinical Psychology, 25*, 294–295.

Gilbert, L. A., Deutsch, C. J., & Strahan, R. F. (1978). Feminine and masculine dimensions of the typical, desirable, and ideal woman and man. *Sex Roles, 4*, 767–778.

Gioe, V. J. (1975). *Cognitive modification and positive group experience as a treatment for depression*. Unpublished doctoral dissertation, Temple University, Philadelphia, PA.

Greenberger, D., & Padesky, C. (1995). *Mind over mood: Change how you feel by changing the way you think*. New York: Guilford Press.

Greene, B. & Blanchard, E. B. (1994). Cognitive therapy for irritable bowel syndrome. *Journal of Consulting and Clinical Psychology, 62*, 576–582.

Greenwald, E., Leitenberg, H., Cado, S., & Tarran, M. (1990). Childhood sexual abuse: Long-term effects on psychological and sexual functioning in a non-clinical and non-student sample of adult women. *Child Abuse and Neglect, 14*, 503–513.

Guthrie, E., Creed, F., Dawson, E., & Tomenson, B. (1991). A controlled trial of psychological treatment for the irritable bowel syndrome. *Gastroenterology, 100*, 450–457.

Hammen, C. (1988). Depression and personal cognitions about personal stressful life events. In L. B. Alloy (Ed.), *Cognitive processes in depression*. New York: Guilford Press.

Harvey, R. F., Hinton, R. A., Gunary, R. M., & Barry, R. E. (1989). Individual and group hypnotherapy in treatment of refractory irritable bowel syndrome. *Lancet, 1*, 424–425.

Hawton, K., Salkovskis, P. M., Kirk, J. W., et al. (Eds.). (1989). *Cognitive-behavioral approaches to adult psychological disorder: A practical guide*. Oxford, UK: Oxford University Press.

Heaton, K. W., O'Donnell, L. J. D., Braddon, F. E. M., Mountford, R. A., Hughes, A. O., & Cripps, P. J. (1992). Symptoms of irritable bowel syndrome in a British urban community: Consulters and nonconsulters. *Gastroenterology, 102,* 1962–1967.

Heimberg, R. G., & Becker, R. E. (1984). *Cognitive-behavioral treatment of social phobia in a group setting.* Albany: State University of New York.

Hollon, S. D., & Shaw, B. F. (1979). Group cognitive therapy for depressed patients. In A. T. Beck, A. J. Rush, B. F. Shaw, & G. Emery *Cognitive therapy of depression* (pp. 328–353). New York: Guilford Press.

Holtzworth-Munroe, A., & Jacobson, N. (1991). Behavioral marital therapy. In A. S. Gurman & D. P. Kniskern (Eds.), *Handbook of family therapy* (Vol. II). New York: Brunner/Mazel.

Holzman, A. D., & Turk, D. C. (1986). *Pain management: A handbook of psychological treatment approaches.* Elmsford, NY: Pergamon Press.

Jack, J. C. (1991). *Silencing the self: Women and depression.* New York: Harper Perennial.

Jack, J. C., & Dill, D. (1992). The Silencing the Self Scale: Schemas of intimacy associated with depression in women. *Psychology of Women Quarterly, 16,* 97–106.

Janoff-Bulman, R. (1979). Characterological versus behavioral self-blame: Inquiries into depression and rape. *Journal of Personality and Social Psychology, 37,* 1798–1809.

Keefe, F. J., Beaupré, P. M., & Gil, K. M. (1996). Group therapy for patients with chronic pain. In R. J. Gatchel & D. C. Turk (Eds.), *Psychological approaches to pain management: A practitioner's handbook* (pp. 259–282). New York: Guilford Press.

Kellow, J. E., Gill, R. C., & Wingate, D. L. (1990). Prolonged ambulant recordings of small bowel motility demonstrate abnormalities in the irritable bowel syndrome. *Gastroenterology, 98,* 1208–1218.

Kelly, J. A., O'Brien, C. G., & Hosford, R. (1981). Sex roles and social skills: Considerations of interpersonal adjustment. *Psychology of Women Quarterly, 5,* 758–766.

Kirmayer, L. J., & Robbins, J. M. (1991). Functional somatic syndromes. In L. J. Kirmayer & J. M. Robbins (Eds.), *Current concepts of somatization.* Washington, DC: American Psychiatric Association Press.

Klass, E. T. (1990). Guilt, shame and embarrassment: Cognitive-behavioral approaches. In I. T. Leitenberg (Ed.), *Handbook of social anxiety* (pp. 34–52). New York: Plenum Press.

Kleinplatz, P., Mccarrey, M., & Kateb, C. (1992). The impact of gender role identity on women's self-esteem, lifestyle satisfaction and conflict. *Canadian Journal of Behavioural Science, 23,* 333–347.

Kovacs, M., & Beck, A. T. (1978). Maladaptive cognitive structures in depression. *American Journal of Psychiatry, 135,* 525–533.

Lange, A. J., & Jakubowski, P. (1976). *Responsible assertive behavior: Cognitive-behavioral procedures for trainers.* Champaign, IL: Research Press.

Laws, A. (1993). Does a history of sexual abuse in childhood play a role in women's medical problems? *Journal of Women's Health, 2,* 165–172.

Lazarus, R. S., & Folkman, S. (1984). *Stress, appraisal and coping.* New York: Springer.

Lechner, M. E., Vogel, M. E., Garcia-Shelton, L. M., Leichter, J. L., & Steibel, K. R. (1993). Self-reported medical problems among adult female survivors of childhood sexual abuse. *Journal of Family Practice, 36,* 633–638.

Leserman, J., Drossman, D. A., Li, Z., Toomey, T. C., Nachman, G., & Glogau, L. (1996). Sexual and physical abuse history in gastroenterology practice: How types of abuse impact health status. *Psychosomatic Medicine, 58,* 4–15.

Levy, R. L., Cain, K. C., Jarriett, M., & Heitkemper, M. M. (1997). The relationship between daily life stress and gastrointestinal symptoms of women with irritable bowel syndrome. *Journal of Behavioral Medicine, 20,* 177–193.

Lewinsohn, P. M., & Graf, M. (1973). Pleasant activities and depression. *Journal of Consulting and Clinical Psychology, 41,* 261–268.

Lips, H. M. (1997). *Sex and gender: An introduction.* Mountain View, CA: Mayfield.

Long, W. O. (1991). Gender role conditioning and women's self-concept. *Journal of Humanistic Education and Development, 30,* 19–29.

Longstreth, G. F., & Wolde-Tsadik, G. (1993). Irritable bowel–type symptoms in HMO examinees: Prevalence, demographics, and clinical correlates. *Digestive Disease Science, 38,* 1581–1589.

Lott, B. L. (1991). Dual natures of learned behaviors: The challenge to feminist psychology. In R. T. Hare-Mustin & J. Marecek (Eds.), *Making a difference: Psychology and the construction of gender.* New Haven, CT: Yale University Press.

Lynch, P. M., & Zamble, E. (1989). A controlled behavioral treatment study of irritable bowel syndrome. *Behavior Therapy, 20,* 509–523.

MacDonald, A. J., & Bouchier, P. A. (1980). Non-organic gastro-intestinal illness: A medical and psychiatric study. *British Journal of Psychiatry, 136,* 1276–1283.

Major, B. (1987). Gender, justice, and the psychology of entitlement. In P. Shaver & C. Hendrick (Eds), *Sex and gender review of personality and social psychology.* Newbury Park, CA: Sage.

Markus, H., Crane, M., Bernstein, S., & Siladi, R. (1982). Self-schemas and gender. *Journal of Personality and Social Psychology, 42,* 38–50.

Mayou, R. (1989). Invited review: A typical chest pain. *Journal of Psychosomatic Research, 33,* 393–406.

Melzack, R., & Wall, P. D. (1965). Pain mechanisms: A new theory. *Science, 150,* 971–980.

Miller, J. B. (1987). *Toward a new psychology of women.* Boston: Beacon Press.

Moldofsky, H., & Lue, F. (1993). Disordered sleep, pain, fatigue, and gastrointestinal symptoms in fibromyalgia, chronic fatigue and irritable bowel syndromes. In H. E. Raybould & E. A. Mayer (Eds.), *Pain research and clinical management*. Amsterdam: Elsevier Science Publications.

Neff, D. F., & Blanchard, E. B. (1987). A multi-component treatment for irritable bowel syndrome. *Behavior Therapy, 18,* 70–83.

Neimeyer, R., & Feixas, G. (1990). The role of homework and skill acquisition in the outcome of group cognitive therapy for depression. *Behavior Therapy, 21,* 281–292.

Newman, C. S. (1994). Understanding clients' resistance: Methods for enhancing motivation to change. *Cognitive Behavioral Practice, 1,* 47–70.

Padesky, C. A., & Greenberger, D. (1995). *Clinician's guide to "Mind Over Mood."* New York: Guilford Press.

Payne, A., & Blanchard, E. G. (1995). A controlled comparison of cognitive therapy and self-help support groups in the treatment of irritable bowel syndrome. *Journal of Consulting and Clinical Psychology, 63,* 779–786.

Pyke, S. W. (1985). Androgyny: An integration. *Journal of Women's Studies, 8,* 529–539.

Resick, P. (1985). Sex role considerations for the behavior therapist. In M. Hersen & A. Bellack (Eds.), *Handbook of clinical behavior therapy with adults*. New York: Plenum Press.

Rimsza, M. E., Berg, R. A., & Locke, C. (1988). Sexual abuse: Somatic and emotional reactions. *Child Abuse and Neglect, 12,* 201–208.

Rolland, J. S. (1994). In sickness and in health: The impact of illness on couples' relationships. *Journal of Marital and Family Therapy, 20,* 327–347.

Rose, E. D., Tolman, R., & Tallant, S. (1985). Group process in cognitive-behavioral therapy. *Behavior Therapist, 8,* 71–75.

Rumsey, N. (1991). Group stress management programmes v. pharmacological treatment in the treatment of the irritable bowel syndrome. In K. W. Keaton, F. Creed, & N. L. M. Goeting (Eds.), *Current approaches towards confident management of irritable bowel syndrome*. Lyme Regis, UK: Lyme Regis Printing Company.

Rush, A. J., & Watkins, J. T. (1981). Group versus individual cognitive therapy: A pilot study. *Cognitive Therapy and Research, 5,* 95–103.

Safran, J. D., & Segal, Z. V. (1990). *Interpersonal process in cognitive therapy*. New York: Basic Books.

Safran, J. D., Segal, Z. V., Shaw, B. F., & Vallis, T. M. (1990). Patient selection for short-term cognitive therapy. In J. D. Safran & Z. V. Segal (Eds.), *Interpersonal process in cognitive therapy*. New York: Basic Books.

Salkovskis, P. (1989). Somatic disorders. In K. Hawton, P. M. Salkovskis, J. W. Kirk, et al. (Eds.), *Cognitive behavioral approaches to adult psychological disorder: A practical guide*. Oxford, UK: Oxford University Press.

Salkovskis, P. (1992). The cognitive-behavioral approach. In F. Creed, R. Mayou, & A. Hopkins (Eds.), *Medical symptoms not explained by organic disease*. London: Royal College of Physicians and Surgeons & Royal College of Physicians.

Salkovskis, P. (1995). *Assessment and treatment of somatic patients*. Workshop, Toronto, Canada.

Salkovskis P., & Warwick, H. M. C. (1986). Morbid preoccupations, health anxiety, and reassurance: A cognitive-behavioral approach to hypochondriasis. *Behaviour Research and Therapy, 24,* 597–602.

Sandler, R. S. (1990). Epidemiology of irritable bowel syndrome in the United States. *Gastroenterology, 99,* 409–415.

Sandler, R. S., Drossman, D. A., Nathan, H. P., & McKee, D. C. (1984). Symptom complaints and health care seeking behavior in subjects with bowel dysfunction. *Gastroenterology, 87,* 314–318.

Sandmaier, M. (1991, February). What's stress got to do with it? *Working Woman,* p. 90.

Sears, R. R. (1970). Relation of early socialization to self-concepts and gender role in middle childhood. *Child Development, 41,* 267–289.

Shaef, A. (1985). *Women's reality.* Minneapolis: Winston Press.

Sharpe, M., Peveler, R., & Mayou, R. (1992). The psychological treatment of patients with functional somatic symptoms: A practical guide. *Journal of Psychosomatic Research, 36,* 515–529.

Shaw, B. F. (1979). A comparison of cognitive therapy and behavior therapy in the treatment of depression. *Journal of Consulting and Clinical Psychology, 45,* 543–551.

Shaw, G., Srivastaa, E. D., Sadlier, M., Swann, P., James, J. Y., & Rhodes, J. (1991). Stress management for irritable bowel syndrome: A controlled trial. *Digestion, 50,* 36–42.

Spielberger, C. D. (1985). Assessment of trait and state anxiety: Conceptual and methodological issues. *Southern Psychologist, 2,* 6–16.

Steiner-Adair, K. (1986). The body politic: Normal female adolescent development and the development of eating disorders. *Journal of the American Academy of Psychoanalysis, 14,* 95–114.

Svedlund, J. (1983). Psychotherapy in irritable bowel syndrome: A controlled outcome study. *Acta Psychiatrica Scandinavica (Supplementum), 306,* 1–86.

Talley, N. J. (1996). Abuse and functional gastrointestinal disorders: What is the link and should we care? *Gastroenterology, 110,* 1301–1304.

Talley, N. J., Boyce, P. M., & Jones, M. (1997). Predictors of health care seeking for irritable bowel syndrome: A population based study. *Gut, 41,* 394–398.

Talley, N. J., Fett, S. L., Zinsmeister, A. R., & Melton, L. J. (1994). Gastrointestinal tract symptoms and self-report abuse: A population-based study. *Gastroenterology, 107,* 1040–1049.

Talley, N. J., Zinsmeister, A. R., Van Dyke, C., & Melton, L. I. (1991). Epidemiology of colonic symptoms and the irritable bowel syndrome. *Gastroenterology, 101,* 927–934.

Taylor, F., & Marshall, W. (1977). Experimental analysis of a cognitive behavioral therapy for depression. *Cognitive Therapy and Research, 5,* 59–72.

Thompson, W. G., Dotevall, G., Drossman, D. A., Heaton, K. W., & Kruis, W. (1989). Irritable bowel syndrome: Guidelines for the diagnosis. *Gastroenterology International, 2,* 92–95.

Thompson, W. G., Heaton, K. W., Smyth, T., & Smyth, C. (1996). Irritable bowel syndrome: The view from general practice [Abstract]. *Gastroenterology, 110,* 705.

Timko, C., Striegel-Moore, R. H., Silberstein, L. R., & Rodin, J. (1987). Femininity/masculinity and disordered eating in women: How are they related? *International Journal of Eating Disorders, 6,* 701–712.

Toner, B. B. (1994). Cognitive-behavioral treatment of functional somatic syndromes: Integrating gender issues. *Cognitive and Behavioral Practice, 1,* 157–178.

Toner, B. B., & Akman, D. (1999). *Gender issues in irritable bowel syndrome.* Unpublished manuscript.

Toner, B. B., Ali, A., Stuckless, N., Weaver, H., Akman, D. E., Tang, T. N. Quattrochocchi, D., & Esplen, M. J. (1999, August). *Development of a gender role socialization scale for women.* Paper presented at the Annual Meeting of the American Psychological Association, Boston.

Toner, B. B., Garfinkel, P. E., & Jeejeebhoy, K. N. (1990). Psychological factors in irritable bowel syndrome. *Canadian Journal of Psychiatry, 35,* 158–161.

Toner, B. B., Garfinkel, P. E., Jeejeebhoy, K. N., Scher, H., Shulhan, D., & DiGasbarro, I. (1990). Self-schema in irritable bowel syndrome. *Psychosomatic Medicine, 52,* 149–155.

Toner, B. B., Koyama, E., Garfinkel, P. E., Jeejeebhoy, K., & DiGasbarro, I. (1992). Social desirability and irritable bowel syndrome. *International Journal of Psychiatry in Medicine, 22,* 99–103.

Toner, B. B., Segal, Z. V., Emmott, S., Myran, D., Ali, A., DiGasbarro, I., & Stuckless, N. (1998). Cognitive-behavioral group therapy for patients with irritable bowel syndrome. *International Journal of Group Psychotherapy, 38,* 215–243.

Toner, B. B., Stuckless, N., Ali, A., Downie, F., Emmott, S., & Akman, D. (1998a). The development of a cognitive scale for functional bowel disorders. *Psychosomatic Medicine, 60,* 492–497.

Toner, B. B., Stuckless, N., Ali, A., Downie, F. P., Emmott, S. D., & Akman, D. E. (1998b). A cognitive scale for functional bowel disorders: An exploration of themes. In H. Goebell, G. Holtmann, & N. J. Talley (Eds.), *Functional dyspepsia and irritable bowel syndrome: Concepts and controversies.* Lancaster, UK: Kluwer.

Turk, D. C., Meichenbaum, D., & Genest, M. (1978). *Pain and behavioral medicine: A cognitive-behavioral perspective.* New York: Guilford Press.

Van Dulmen, A. M., Fennis, J. F., & Bleijenberg, G. (1996). Cognitive-behavioral group therapy for irritable bowel syndrome: Effects and long-term follow-up. *Psychosomatic Medicine, 58,* 508–514.

Voirol, M. W., & Hipolito, J. (1987). Anthropo-analytical relaxation in irritable bowel syndrome: Results 40 months later. *Schweizerische Medizinische Wochenschrift, 117,* 1117–1119.

Vollmer, A., & Blanchard, E. B. (1998). Controlled comparison of individual versus group cognitive therapy for irritable bowel syndrome. *Behavior Therapy, 29,* 19–33.

Walker, E. A., Gelfand, A. N., Gelfand, M. D., Koss, M. P., & Katon, W. J. (1995). Medical and psychiatric symptoms in women gastroenterology clinic patients with histories of sexual victimization. *General Hospital Psychiatry, 97*, 108–118.

Walker, E. A., Katon, W. J., Harrop-Griffiths, J., Holm, L., Russo, J., & Hickock, L. R. (1988). Relationship of chronic pelvic pain to psychiatric diagnoses and childhood sexual abuse. *American Journal of Psychiatry, 145*, 75–80.

Walker, E. A., Katon, W. J., Roy-Burne, P. P., Jemelka, R. P., & Russo, J. (1993). Histories of sexual victimization in patients with irritable bowel syndrome or inflammatory bowel disease. *American Journal of Psychiatry, 150*, 1502–1506.

Warwick, H. M. C., & Salkovskis, P. (1990). Hypochondriasis. *Behaviour Research and Therapy, 28*, 105–118.

Whitehead, W. E. (1998). Is a history of abuse linked to the aetiology and course of functional dyspepsia and irritable bowel syndrome? No. In H. Goebell, G. Holtmann, & N. J. Talley (Eds.), *Functional dyspepsia and irritable bowel syndrome: Concepts and controversies.* Lancaster, UK: Kluwer.

Whitehead, W. E., Bosmajian, L., Zonderman, A. B., Costa, P. T., Jr., & Schuster M. M. (1988). Symptoms of psychologic distress associated with irritable bowel syndrome: Comparison of community and medical clinic samples. *Gastroenterology, 95*, 709–714.

Whitehead, W. E., Cheskin, L. J., Heller, B. R., Robinson, C., Crowel, M. D., Benjamin, C., & Schuster, M. (1990). Evidence for exacerbation of irritable bowel syndrome during menses. *Gastroenterology, 98*, 1485–1489.

Whorwell, P. J., McCallum, M., Creed, F. H., et al. (1986). Non-colonic features of irritable bowel syndrome. *Gut, 27*, 37–40.

Whorwell, P. J., Prior, A., & Colgan, S. M. (1987). Hypnotherapy in severe irritable bowel syndrome: Further experience. *Gut, 28*, 423–425.

Whorwell, P. J., Prior, A., & Faragher, E. B. (1984). Controlled trial of hypnotherapy in the treatment of severe refractory irritable bowel syndrome. *Lancet, 2*, 1232–1233.

Williams, J. M. R. (1992). *The psychological treatment of depression.* New York: Routledge.

Wise, T. N., Cooper, J. N., & Ahmed, M. D. (1982). The efficacy of group therapy for patients with irritable bowel syndrome. *Psychosomatics, 23*, 465–469.

Worell, J., & Remer, P. (1992). *Feminist perspectives in therapy: An empowerment model for women.* Toronto: Wiley.

Young, S. J., Alpers, D. H., Norland, C. C., & Woodruff, R. A. (1976). Psychiatric illness and the irritable bowel syndrome. *Gastroenterology, 70*, 162–166.

Index

"t" indicates a table

Ingram Content Group UK Ltd.
Milton Keynes UK
UKHW041806090723
424689UK00007B/22

9 781572 301351